'As far as the stimulant effect is con   say, a Red Bull.'

'Forget coffee and chocolate . . . there are far more natural ways to feel good.' *Sunday Express*

'On my last book tour I left strong men standing. That was due, I'm sure, to the supplements. I continue to consult Patrick Holford for optimal energy.' *Shirley Conran*

'After being "on the go" for more than 36 hours I was in no fit state to drive so I took a combination of your natural stimulants about 20 minutes before I set off. Being fairly sceptical I wasn't expecting amazing results. However, I was amazed! Within minutes I felt wide awake, alert and ready for action. This state lasted a good five hours with NO discernable side effects. I would recommend them over caffeine any day.' *IG*

'I've been using the natural stimulants you recommend with great joy; I think they're the BEST stimulants I've ever taken. In fact one of the things I've really liked about them is that they are so mellow. You don't feel that you've taken a stimulant at all, you just feel happily alert. What you are doing is genuinely groundbreaking.' *Sally K*

'After a five-mile run and sumptuous dinner I was concerned about staying awake on a $2^1/_2$-hour drive home, until I discovered the herbs and nutrients you recommend. Instead of having coffee I took these. For the whole drive I was as perky and bright as a button. When I reached my destination my friends were ready for bed but I was wide awake.' *NH*

NATURAL HIGHS
energy

25 ways to increase your energy

PATRICK HOLFORD
& DR HYLA CASS

PIATKUS

Copyright © 2003 by Patrick Holford & Dr Hyla Cass

First published in 2003 by
Judy Piatkus (Publishers) Limited
5 Windmill Street
London W1T 2JA
e-mail: info@piatkus.co.uk

The moral right of the authors has been asserted

A catalogue record for this book is available from the British Library

ISBN 0 7499 2334 2

Edited by Barbara Kiser
Text design by Paul Saunders

This book has been printed on paper manufactured with respect for the
environment using wood from managed sustainable resources

Typeset by Palimpsest Book Production Limited, Polmont, Stirlingshire
Printed and bound in Great Britain by William Clowes, Beccles, Suffolk

Contents

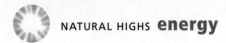

Acknowledgements

W E WOULD LIKE TO THANK Oscar Ichazo for his generosity in letting us share the Diakath Breathing exercise and Doors of Compensation with you; Caroline Vellacott for her help with the chapters on yoga and meditation; Susannah Lawson for her help with the chapter on t'ai chi; and most of all Shane Heaton for his help in researching and editing. We are also indebted to our publishers, and especially Gill Bailey, Penny Phillips, and Barbara Kiser for her careful editing.

Introduction

ARE YOU TIRED of being tired? Do you wake up needing something to get you going, or run out of energy before the day is through? If so, you're not alone. Seven in every ten of us complain of the same thing – a kind of general exhaustion. So we guzzle coffee, tea and fizzy drinks, and hit the sugar or cigarettes, all to boost our flagging reserves of energy. Sad to say, but our attempts don't last very long.

If you want to thrive in the speeded-up, round-the-clock 21st century, you need new ways to keep you feeling energised. That's what this book is about – how to build a new way of living, at home and at work, that actually works. This book gives you 25 simple techniques to boost your energy levels. Some are nutritional (like tyrosine and rhodiola), some are psychological (like how to think positive and live in the present), some are physical (like Psychocalisthenics and top tips for sleeping) and some are environmental (like using sound and smell). For more information on these topics, read our book, *Natural Highs*.

Put these techniques together and you have a recipe for instant energy. And it works, as Ian, a website programmer, found. 'I was amazed! Within minutes I felt wide awake, alert and ready for action. This state lasted a good five hours with NO discernable side effects.' Ian has now given coffee the thumbs down. You can get off the caffeine carousel, too, by putting these simple techniques into practice in your life.

Wishing you high energy living.

Patrick Holford and Dr Hyla Cass

1

Amino Acids Can Keep You Alert

EVER HAD ONE of those flat, down days that have you moaning for something, anything, to give you that yearned-for shot of energy? Most pick-me-ups are beguiling, but ineffective. Going to work on a supplement of amino acids, however, can give you real mental and physical energy and enthusiasm, and let you leave the lethargy behind.

Amino acids are the building blocks of protein. Some of them are essential for energy because they also provide the basic materials for the brain's neurotransmitters – the chemical messengers that allow the trillions of cells in the brain to

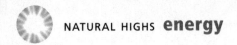

communicate with one another, so effectively controlling how
you think and feel.

The key stimulatory amino acids are tyrosine and phenylalanine. They're specifically involved in enhancing mental
alertness, raising mood and boosting energy, mental performance and memory. If you are low in phenylalanine or tyrosine,
you may feel tired and sluggish, have trouble concentrating and
find it hard to get out of bed in the morning. A dose of either
can really get you motivated and ready for action.

Why They're Good

We lump these two amino acids together because phenylalanine
is converted into tyrosine in the body. The tyrosine is then made
into the stimulating brain chemicals dopamine, adrenalin and
noradrenalin. It's in this way that these two amino acids can have
such a positive effect on your mood, motivation and energy level.

More energy

Caffeine works, in large part, by stimulating dopamine, adrenalin and noradrenalin production. So tyrosine and phenylalanine can give you a similar lift, but without the sudden drop afterwards typical of caffeine and other stimulants. If you're gasping for a caffeine boost, taking phenylalanine or tyrosine instead, directly under the tongue, can give you the kick you want without the downside. Further, they can help you get off energy-sapping stimulants such as cigarettes, caffeine and alcohol altogether, as they are instrumental in restoring normal brain chemistry.

Better mood and motivation

Both of these amino acids can raise the levels of dopamine and other mood-enhancing chemicals in the brain such as endorphins. Because they're turned into adrenalin and noradrenalin in the body, they can also increase your motivation and mental alertness, and improve your stress tolerance.

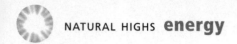

Better performance under stress

While a certain level of stress can motivate us to perform better, when we're chronically or excessively stressed our physical and mental performance can deteriorate rapidly. Clearly, this presents problems for the military, and so a team of American researchers were very interested to find that giving tyrosine to soldiers in stressful conditions of extreme temperatures or intense physical activity, over prolonged periods of time, dramatically improved both their physical and mental endurance.

This finding was confirmed recently in Holland, where 21 cadets were put through a demanding one-week combat training course. Ten received a drink supplying 2g of tyrosine a day, while the others were given an identical drink without the tyrosine. Those on tyrosine consistently outperformed their peers, both mentally and physically, throughout the course.[1]

Where to Find Them

As amino acids are the building blocks of protein, they are present in all protein-rich foods, such as fish, dairy products, beans, meat, lentils, tofu, nuts and seeds. However, some people need more than they can get from diet alone, so supplements of tyrosine and phenylalanine are widely available in health food stores.

How and When to Take Them and How Much

Dopamine, adrenalin and noradrenalin become depleted when you're stressed or overusing stimulants such as caffeine and nicotine. At these times you need phenylalanine and tyrosine more than ever. While these two amino acids have very similar effects on your mood, motivation and energy levels, there are slight differences in their other effects that can help you decide which one to try.

Because tyrosine is made in the body from phenylalanine, it usually acts more rapidly when supplemented, as it's one step nearer to becoming the energising neurotransmitters dopamine, noradrenalin and adrenalin. Tyrosine is also used in the production of thyroid hormones, known to control energy levels and manage your metabolic rate. When your thyroid function is low, so is your energy level.

While this may sound like tyrosine is the way to go,

remember that your body makes it out of phenylalanine anyway, and some people find phenylalanine more effective than tyrosine for stimulation. Phenylalanine also has other actions that tyrosine does not, such as helping control appetite and acting as a pain reliever.

Whichever one works best for you, take it on an empty stomach (for example, first thing in the morning) because amino acids in protein foods compete for absorption with each other.

The best form of phenylalanine to take is DL-phenylalanine, or DLPA for short. The effective dose is usually 500 to 1000mg. For quick absorption, open the capsule and put the powder under your tongue. Watch your energy and mood go up. Also helpful are 50mg of vitamin B6 and 500mg of vitamin C to enhance phenylalanine's conversion to tyrosine. You can take more DLPA later in the day if needed, but not too close to bedtime.

Taking 500 to 1000mg of tyrosine on an empty stomach first thing in the morning can really lift your motivation and energy level for the rest of the day.

Any Precautions?

As these amino acids naturally occur in your diet, they are generally safe. However, when supplementing, too much phenylalanine or tyrosine can cause overstimulation, anxiety, insomnia and elevated blood pressure in some people. If this happens, lower the dose, and if symptoms persist, stop taking it altogether. For these reasons, if you already have high blood pressure or a history of mania, this may not be the best natural stimulant for you. Neither amino acid should be taken with MAO inhibitors, a kind of antidepressant involving certain food restrictions; by phenylketonurics (people who have a metabolic disorder); by those with malignant melanomas (they increase sunlight sensitivity); or during pregnancy and breastfeeding.

2

Aromatherapy Awakeners

A CENTURY AGO, SMELLING SALTS were used to jolt swooning women up and out of their woozy condition. Nowadays, we may not rely on our noses to help us regain consciousness, but we can use our sensitivity to smell to keep us constantly wide awake, watchful and alert.

Aromatherapy is the selective use of aromas from certain essential oils. These smells are carried directly by the olfactory nerves to the brain, where they have a direct effect on how we think and feel. Certain essential oils can increase your energy and alertness.

Why They're Good For You

As far back as the 1920s, Italian psychiatrists Giovanni Gatti and Renato Cayola found that the scents of angelica, cardamom, cinnamon, clove, fennel, lemon and ylang ylang had a stimulating effect. More recently, research in the US has proved that peppermint and eucalyptus also stimulate the brain and promote alertness. Meanwhile, in Japan, Dr Shizuo Torii of the Toho University School of Medicine in Tokyo showed that some of these fragrances increased the incidence of beta waves in the brain. Beta waves are the pattern of brain activity that is associated with alert attention. His research also showed that basil, jasmine, sage, patchouli and black pepper act as stimulants.

Stimulation without stress

While these oils wake you up and keep you alert, they don't stimulate the adrenal glands, putting you into a stressful state. They actually reduce stress and help to promote a more relaxed state of alert attention. They also relieve drowsiness and irritability and, in some people, lessen or prevent headaches.

Improved work performance

Dr Torii has found that these oils work by arousing the nervous system, which also controls breathing and blood pressure, and that they can help to keep you alert. This was confirmed by research at the University of Cincinnati testing the effects of essential oils on alertness by giving people a stress test, involving a 40-minute task based on identifying patterns on a computer. Those working in rooms scented with peppermint had many more correct answers than people working in unscented rooms, and were able to perform better for longer. In another study at the Rensselaer Polytechnic Institute in New York, workers were more effective at achieving specific targets they set for themselves when their offices were scented – even when they didn't think the scents were having any effect.

Stimulating essential oils can improve your performance in the workplace by promoting a more consistent level of alert attention, without promoting stress.

Relaxed and stimulated

Some fragrances are both relaxing and stimulating. These include jasmine, musk, patchouli, rose, sandalwood, vanilla and ylang ylang. While not as stimulating as, say, lemon, peppermint or eucalyptus, they do keep you alert and are good to use when stressed at work.

How and When to Take Them and How Much

Use good-quality, pure essential oils. The complex blend of chemicals in the natural fragrances can't be duplicated in the laboratory, so avoid synthetic versions.

The best oils for stimulation include cinnamon, eucalyptus, lemon, patchouli, peppermint and sage. These invigorate the senses and encourage natural alertness. They are great to use at work. Many businesses in Japan place fragrances in their air-conditioning systems. Citrus is often used in the morning to awaken, while peppermint is used in factories to reduce stress, and ylang-ylang is often used towards the end of the working day for its calming effects. Scent your home or workspace using aromatherapy burners or diffusers, or simply sprinkle drops on the carpet, curtains or even your own clothing.

For an invigorating massage, you need to blend one of the

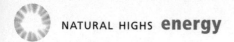

stimulating essential oils mentioned on page 13 with a 'carrier' oil (such as sweet almond oil, available in health food stores). Use 5ml of essence to 115ml of carrier oil. Make your own energising perfume by mixing your favourite essential oils in a small amount of carrier oil just as you do for massage. For bath oils, blend 5ml of essence with 60ml of carrier oil.

Where to Find Them

A variety of essential oil blends designed to keep you alert can be found in most health food stores. Choose pure essential oil blends that contain the stimulating oils listed on page 13.

Any Precautions?

A small number of people are sensitive to certain oils. You can test yourself by putting a drop on your skin. If your skin becomes red or itchy, avoid that essential oil.

3

Ashwagandha – India's Ginseng

WHEN YOU'RE COMPLETELY HAPPY and content, you don't stop to think about it – you just waltz buoyantly along. The same is true of feeling energised. Normal, healthy levels of vitality go unnoticed; it's only when you begin to wilt that you realise you were previously surfing a wave of energy and vitality. If you long to feel ceaselessly, naturally alive without having to bother about where you can get your next burst of energy, try ashwagandha.

Known as 'Indian ginseng', ashwagandha (*Withania somnifera*) is a small evergreen shrub and a member of the night-

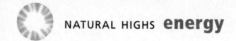

shade family, though without the poisonous attributes. It grows in dry areas of India and as far west as Israel and the Mediterranean, and has been used for thousands of years in traditional Indian Ayurvedic medicine to treat stress-related ailments. Now ashwagandha is increasingly being integrated into Western herbal practice. It is a well-known adaptogen that tones and normalises bodily functions and renders the body more resistant to stress (more on this on page 17). It's also a recognised aphrodisiac. The word ashwagandha literally means 'the sweat of a horse', suggesting that one who takes it would have the strength and sexual vitality of a horse! All parts of the plant, though especially the root, are used medicinally.

Why It's Good

Ashwagandha has been used for centuries by practitioners of Ayurvedic medicine to help people who want to safely and naturally increase their stamina, energy level, mental clarity and focus. Researchers have been studying ashwagandha since the early 1960s, and chemical analysis has revealed that it contains phytonutrient compounds such as withanolides, glycosides and several different alkaloids, thought to have anti-stress, sedative, anti-tumour, anti-inflammatory and anti-fungal properties. This versatile herb gives you more energy while calming your stress response by reducing high levels of the stress hormone cortisol.

An all-round star

As I've mentioned, ashwagandha is an adaptogen. These are substances that enhance and regulate the body's ability to withstand stress and increase its general performance, helping the whole body to resist disease. As such, ashwagandha is claimed to boost strength, increase stamina and relieve fatigue, enhance sexual energy and rejuvenate the body, strengthen the immune system, speed recovery from chronic illness, strengthen sickly children, soothe and calm without producing drowsiness, clarify the mind and improve memory, and even slow down the ageing process! In a study comparing this herb with panax ginseng, another well known adaptogen, ashwagandha was found to be superior in improving physical and mental function.

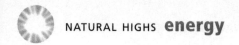

Boosts your thyroid

Because your thyroid gland controls your metabolic rate – the rate at which you produce energy – a sluggish or sub-clinically underactive thyroid is a sure road to poor mental and physical energy. Ashwagandha increases thyroid hormone levels, thus speeding up the metabolism, raising body temperature, improving circulation and getting your fire burning again.

Energising but calming

Ashwagandha has a sedative effect on the central nervous system, and can enhance the effect of any other central-nervous-system sedatives (such as alcohol) that are taken at the same time. This should be kept in mind if you need to be especially alert.

Increases brain power

Ashwagandha can also enhance memory and cognition due to its antioxidant effect and ability to increase acetylcholine receptor activity in the brain. Acetylcholine is a neurotransmitter, or chemical messenger, in the brain that's involved in memory. If the receptors in your brain 'listen' for it more, as ashwagandha appears to make them do, you can enjoy greater mental acuity, a clearer memory and heightened alertness.

How and When to Take It and How Much

Ashwagandha tea can be made by simmering a teaspoon of the dried powdered root in a litre of water for 15 minutes. Three cups a day is recommended. The tincture dosage is 2 to 4ml (0.5 to 1 tsp) daily in a little water. However, the most convenient way to take ashwagandha is in capsules of extract and/or dried whole root powder: 300mg of standardised extract, containing 1.5 per cent withanolides, two to three times daily, is recommended. See which dose works best for you, as the correct dose depends on both your body type and the state of your health.

Where to Find It

Ashwagandha is now available in most health food stores as a tincture or capsules of the dried root powder. Look for standardised extracts that guarantee at least 1.5 per cent of the active ingredient withanolides. Although ashwagandha can be taken alone, it is traditionally combined with other herbs in tonics and natural stimulant formulas to enhance its rejuvenating effects.

Any Precautions?

Botanical safety guidelines in the US and Germany have suggested that taking ashwagandha is not suitable during pregnancy. To date, there have not been any other reports of possible medical contraindications, side effects or potential health hazards. It has been used successfully for the last 3,000 years, and the empirical evidence of the ages speaks for itself. However, there is an argument that no herb should be consumed for long periods of time (more than three months), and that herbs may best be reserved for 'times of need'.

4

B Vitamins for Vitality

IF IT'S A FATIGUE-FIGHTER and stamina-strengthener you're after, B vitamins could be just what you need. Many people don't get enough of these energy-boosting nutrients. Ensuring an optimum supply will keep you so alive and 'ever-ready' that you'll simply never feel like a failing battery in need of constant recharging.

B vitamins are a family of eight different substances, every one essential for making energy. Glucose can't be turned into energy without B1, B2, B3 (niacin) and B5 (pantothenic acid). Fats and proteins can't be used to make energy without B6, B12, folic acid or biotin.

It used to be thought that as long as you ate a reasonable diet, you'd get enough B vitamins. But studies have shown that long-term slight deficiencies gradually result in symptoms such as poor skin condition, anxiety, depression, irritability, but most of all, fatigue. Only one in 10 people have a diet that provides even the basic recommended daily allowance (RDA) levels for all the Bs, let alone the optimal amounts needed to maximise your vitality.

Why They're Good

More energy

In one study at the Institute for Optimum Nutrition, we gave volunteers, many of whom already had a 'well-balanced diet', extra B vitamins in supplement form – often in doses 10 times that of the RDAs, which are the kind of levels now thought to be the ideal intakes of these vitamins. After 6 months, 79 per cent of participants reported a definite improvement in energy, 61 per cent felt physically fitter, and 60 per cent noticed an improvement in their mental alertness and memory. Most people notice a definite increase in energy within 10 days of supplementing B vitamins.

Better concentration

There's no doubt that B vitamins can give your mind and memory a boost too. After all, the brain uses more nutrients than any other part of the body. Our first IQ study, published in *The Lancet* in 1987, gave children multivitamins containing optimal amounts of all the B vitamins. The children on the vitamins had a 10-point increase in IQ compared to those on placebos.[2] Fifteen studies have now confirmed that multivitamins can increase IQ scores. They do this by boosting your powers of concentration and focus. They literally help your brain to work efficiently.

Smoother moods

Due to all this extra energy and improved concentration, you'll have more stable and happier moods. In fact, some of the most common deficiency signs of B vitamins are depression, anxiety and irritability. If you're really deficient, you can even go crazy. B vitamins can smoothe your moods out because they help make neurotransmitters, the brain's natural highs that keep you energised, relaxed and happy.

Improved health

There are a hundred and one other amazing things that B vitamins do for you – from improving your skin to helping you digest your food. B vitamins boost your immune system, prevent headaches and help your body and brain regenerate, keeping you young and bright. They also help to keep your blood sugar level even and are vital for delivering oxygen to the brain.

How and When to Take Them and How Much

Because they are water soluble, B vitamins are simply excreted in your urine if you take in more than you need. But because of this water solubility, and their sensitivity to heat, B vitamins are also easily lost when foods are boiled in water. The best natural sources are therefore fresh fruit and raw vegetables.

To achieve a guaranteed optimal amount you really need to take supplements. This means a high-strength multivitamin or a B complex containing:

B1 (thiamine)	25 to	100mg
B2 (riboflavin)	25 to	100mg
B3 (niacin)	50 to	150mg
B5 (pantothenic acid)	50 to	200mg
B6 (pyridoxine)	50 to	100mg
B12 (cyanocobalamin)	10 to	100mcg
Folic acid	100 to	400mcg
Biotin	25 to	75mcg

Where to Find Them

As far as foods are concerned, the best for B vitamins include fresh fruit and vegetables, as mentioned above. Seeds, nuts

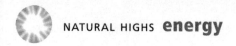

and wholegrains, especially wheatgerm, contain reasonable amounts, as do meat, fish, eggs and dairy produce. But these levels are reduced when the food is cooked or stored for a long time.

As far as supplements are concerned there are many good multivitamins and B complex supplements to choose from in health food stores. Stay away from multivitamins that claim 100 per cent of the RDA – that's too little if you want to maximise your energy levels.

Any Precautions?

There are a few. B6 and B3 can be toxic if a person were to consume several grams – but who would want to do that? If you have enough B2, your urine goes almost fluorescent yellow, especially if you don't drink enough water. But this doesn't constitute a problem.

5

Breathing for Energy

'THE BREATH OF life', 'a breath of fresh air', 'breathing space' . . . Breathing is essential for energy, and not just because we take in oxygen that way. Yet most people use less than a third of their lungs when they breathe. No wonder so many of us feel leaden and exhausted.

Exercise and breathing exercises increase lung capacity, and so help to oxygenate the tissues and improve energy levels. Breathing is something we take for granted, and yet for thousands of years, ancient traditions have used breathing exercises to bring about conscious, healthful changes in the body.

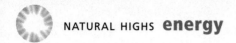

Our breathing is a reflection of our emotions. For example, when we are anxious or afraid, our breathing becomes rapid and shallow. When we are happy and at ease, our breathing is naturally slow and deep. The breath is the link between mind and body. Simply by becoming conscious of your breathing, you can both calm the mind and relax the body. The air we breathe also contains vital energy, known as *prana* or *chi*. By regularly doing the following conscious breathing exercises we can accumulate this energy and revitalise the body and mind.

Diakath Breathing^{sm}

The breathing exercise by Oscar Ichazo, founder of the Arica School, a school of knowledge, uses the diaphragm muscle to guide our breathing pattern so that deep breathing becomes natural and effortless, allowing us to be aware of the Kath^{sm} point during the exercise. You can practice this exercise at any time, while sitting, standing or lying down, and for as long as you like. You can also do it unobtrusively during moments of stress.

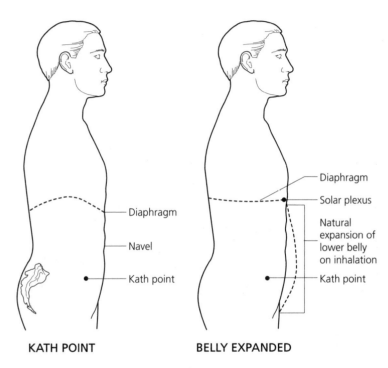

KATH POINT

BELLY EXPANDED

Diakath Breathing

©2002 Oscar Ichazo. Diakath Breathing and Kath are service marks of Oscar Ichazo. Used by permission.

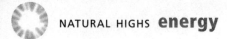

The diaphragm is a dome-shaped muscle attached to the bottom of the rib cage. The Kath is not an anatomical point like the navel, but is the body's centre of equilibrium, located in the lower belly about three finger widths below the navel. When you keep your attention in this point you become aware of your entire body.

How to do It

In Diakath Breathing your lower belly expands from the Kath point as you inhale. The diaphragm muscle expands downwards towards the Kath point. This allows the lungs to fill with air from the bottom to the top. As you exhale, the belly and the diaphragm muscle relax, allowing the lungs to empty from top to bottom. Inhale and exhale through your nose.

1. Sit comfortably, in a quiet place with your spine straight.

2. Focus your attention in your Kath point.

3. Let your belly expand from the Kath point as you inhale slowly and deeply. Feel your diaphragm being pulled down

towards the Kath point, as your lungs fill with air from the bottom to the top.

4. On the exhale, relax both your belly and your diaphragm, emptying your lungs from top to bottom.

5. Repeat at your own pace.

When to do It

- Every morning sit down in a quiet place before breakfast and practise Diakath Breathing for 5 minutes, or 36 breaths.

- Whenever you are stressed throughout the day, check your breathing. Practice Diakath Breathing for nine breaths. This is great to do before an important meeting, or when something has upset you.

6

Caffeine – Give It Up

IT'S A SACRED MORNING RITUAL for millions: wake up and blearily head for the coffee maker. And yes, a cup of the stuff does make you feel better, more energised and alert – for a while, at least. But at what cost, and why?

Dr Peter Rogers, a psychologist at Bristol University, wondered whether coffee actually increases your energy and mental performance, or just relieves symptoms of withdrawal. When he researched this he found that after that first cup of coffee, coffee drinkers don't feel any better than people who never drink coffee. Coffee drinkers just feel better than they did when they woke up.[3] In other words, drinking coffee is highly effective at relieving the symptoms of withdrawal from coffee.

Why It's Bad

Caffeine blocks the receptors for a brain chemical called adenosine, whose function is to stop the release of the motivating neurotransmitters dopamine and adrenalin. With less adenosine activity, levels of dopamine and adrenalin increase, as does alertness and motivation.

But there's a catch. Caffeine is addictive. The more often you have it, the more often you need it. The more you consume caffeine, the more the body and brain become insensitive to the power of its own stimulants, dopamine and adrenalin. You then need more stimulants to feel normal, and keep demanding the body to produce more dopamine and adrenalin. The net result is adrenal exhaustion – an inability to produce these important chemicals of motivation and communication. Apathy, depression, exhaustion and inability to cope set in.

And there's more. Caffeine worsens mental performance. A study published in the *American Journal of Psychiatry* studied 1,500 psychology students and found that more than one coffee a day caused more anxiety, depression, and stress-related medical problems, and lower academic performance.[4] A number of studies have shown that the ability to remember lists of words is made worse by caffeine. According to one researcher, 'Caffeine may have a deleterious effect on the rapid processing of ambiguous or confusing stimuli,' which sounds like a description of modern living!

How much is too much?

Coffee isn't the only source of caffeine. Tea, cola drinks and chocolate all contain caffeine. There's as much in a strong cup of tea as in a regular cup of coffee. Caffeine is also the active ingredient, together with sugar, in most cola and other so-called 'energy' drinks such as Red Bull. Chocolate and green tea also contain caffeine, but much less than these drinks do. For example, a regular coffee contains 50 to 100mg of caffeine – a so-called 'grande' can contain up to 500mg. A cup of tea contains from 20 to 100mg, depending on how strong you have it. Most cola drinks contain around 50mg of caffeine, while the 'energy' drinks go up to 80mg. A cup of green tea or 10 squares of chocolate will give you 20mg.

If you 'have to' have it, you're addicted and therefore having too much. Certainly, when you consume more than 100mg of caffeine there's clear evidence of negative effects.

What's the Alternative?

Coffee contains three stimulants – caffeine, theobromine and theo-phylline. Although caffeine is the strongest, theophylline is known to disturb normal sleep patterns, and theobromine has a similar effect to caffeine, although it is present in much smaller amounts in coffee. So decaffeinated coffee isn't exactly stimulant-free. The most popular stimulant-free alternatives are Caro Extra or Bambu (made with roasted chicory and malted barley), and dandelion coffee (Symingtons or Lanes). The best-tasting alternatives to tea are Rooibosch (red bush) tea with milk, and herb and fruit teas. Drinking very weak tea irregularly is unlikely to be a problem.

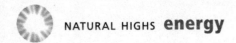

How to Quit

The best way to find out what effect caffeine has on you is to go 'cold turkey' for a trial period of two weeks. You may get withdrawal symptoms for up to three days. These reflect how addicted you've become. After that, you begin to feel perky, have more consistent energy, especially in the mornings, and your health improves. Once you are no longer craving caffeine, the occasional weak cup of tea or very occasional coffee is not a big deal.

One client, Bobbie, serves as a case in point. She was already eating a healthy diet and took a sensible daily programme of vitamin and mineral supplements. She had only two problems: a lack of energy in the morning and occasional headaches. And she had one vice: three cups of coffee a day. After some persuasion, she agreed to stop drinking coffee for one month. To her surprise up went her energy level and the headaches stopped.

7

Chromium – the Energy Balancer

HEALTH IS ONE GREAT BIG BALANCING ACT. A body that's functioning on an even keel provides you with the foundations, strength and stamina to address other aspects of your life that need equalising. Well, it's all very well knowing this, but putting the theory into practice is no piece of cake. Too many of us try to balance out our exhaustion by reaching for the energy boost of a sugar-laden snack.

If you're doing this all the time, it could be a sign that your body's out of kilter. And here's where chromium comes in – the ideal way to help you out of a sticky fix.

Chromium is an essential mineral that helps stabilise energy levels. Typical dietary intakes are far lower than optimal levels, especially for those with weight and energy problems. Here's why.

Because sugar is your main fuel, and it's transported around the body in your blood, stable levels of 'blood sugar' are the key to consistent levels of energy for brain and body alike. Low or unstable blood sugar levels cause many symptoms of low energy, including fatigue, lethargy, drowsiness, depression, poor memory and concentration, anxiety, irritability and, inevitably, cravings for stimulants or sugar to get you out of this mess. Unfortunately, their effects are short lived and you're soon back where you started, or worse. Many people are on this vicious energy roller-coaster ride all day, every day. Chromium is an important part of the solution.

Why It's Good

Blood sugar balance

Chromium can help get you off the blood sugar roller-coaster because it's a vital constituent of glucose tolerance factor. This is a compound produced in the liver that helps the hormone insulin carry glucose from the blood to the cells. Other nutrients are also required for glucose tolerance factor, such as vitamin B3 and the amino acids glycine, glutamic acid and cystine, but chromium is key.

Diabetics, who have seriously compromised blood sugar control, are known to have lower tissue levels of chromium than non-diabetics,[5] and a double-blind crossover study of eight women with blood sugar imbalance confirmed that supplementing 200mcg of chromium a day can stabilise blood sugar levels, improve glucose tolerance and alleviate all hypoglycaemic symptoms within three months.[6]

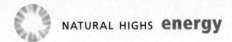

Fat burning

Two further studies carried out at Bemidji State University in Minnesota have shown that chromium supplementation helps to build muscle and burn fat.[7] Chromium can therefore help to turn fat into energy and, if you're exercising, build more muscle. As muscle is metabolically active, it burns fat for you even when you're sleeping, and for many people, less fat means less wastage of energy carrying around that extra baggage.

Energy boost

Many people experience an increase in energy or an increasingly stable level of energy within two or three days of supplementing chromium.

Where to Find It

Chromium is found in wholefoods and is therefore high in brown rice, wholewheat flour, bread and pasta, as well as in other whole grains, beans, nuts and seeds. Asparagus and mushrooms are also rich in chromium. Since it works with insulin to help stabilise your blood sugar level, appetite and weight, the more uneven your blood sugar level, the more chromium you use up. Hence, a sugar and stimulant addict eating refined carbohydrates is most at risk of deficiency. Wheat flour and sugar have 98 per cent of their chromium removed in the refining process – another reason to stay away from refined foods like white bread.

Whether or not you can achieve an optimal intake of chromium from diet alone, even a good diet, is debatable. The average daily dietary intake is below 50mcg, while an optimal intake, certainly for those with energy, weight and blood sugar problems, is around 200mcg. It is therefore wise to take supplements of this fat-burning mineral as well as eating wholefoods.

How and When to Take It and How Much

Body stores of chromium tend to decline with age, so just like many other nutrients, supplementation is more important the older you are.[8]

The best forms of chromium are either picolinate or poly-nicotinate. These forms enable chromium to readily enter the body's cells, where it can then help insulin do its job more effectively. We recommend anyone to supplement around 50 to 100mcg a day, and 200mcg if you're experiencing a low energy level or the symptoms of blood sugar problems, together with a good multivitamin. Chromium is best taken in the morning to help stabilise your blood sugar and energy throughout the day.

Any Precautions?

Chromium is found in two forms in nature – hexavalent and trivalent. Of the two, hexavalent chromium is much more toxic, but luckily for us, it's only found in car bumpers! Trivalent chromium, which is what you get in supplements, has a very low toxicity. An intake of up to 500mcg is certainly considered safe. If you have diabetes, don't take chromium unless under the supervision of your doctor or a nutritionist. It can clearly reduce insulin requirements, so you'll have to monitor your blood sugar level very carefully.

8

Coenzyme-Q – the Undiscovered Vitamin?

IF YOU WANT REAL STAYING POWER, or just the energy to help you sail more smoothly through a demanding day, help could be at hand. A remarkable enzyme, coenzyme-Q, is proving to be a major energy and health booster in all kinds of ways, including increased stamina and improved fitness.

Life depends on enzymes. These control all biochemical reactions in the body – including turning food into energy. Enzymes, in turn, are activated by 'coenzymes' which, more often than not, are vitamins or minerals. Possibly the most important coenzyme for energy production is coenzyme-Q (Co-Q). The discovery that it's present in foods, that tissue levels decline with age, and that levels rise when supplements are taken, has led many nutritional scientists to suspect that Co-Q may be an essential vitamin. Technically, Co-Q can't be classified as a vitamin since it can be made by the body, even if it isn't made in large enough amounts for optimum health and energy. It is therefore a semi-essential nutrient.

Why It's Good

A vital link in the energy-production chain, Co-Q provides the spark, together with oxygen, to keep our energy furnace burning. Co-Q's magical properties lie in its ability to improve the cells' use of oxygen. Our body cells make energy when hydrogen, from carbohydrate, reacts with oxygen, from the air we breathe. Tiny packages of energy called electrons are passed from one atom to the next in what is called the electron-transfer chain. These electrons are highly reactive and need to be very carefully handled. Like nuclear fuel, they're a very dangerous but very potent energy source.

Co-Q has two key roles to play in handling these volatile

electrons. It controls the flow of oxygen, making the production of energy in the electron-transport chain most efficient, and it prevents electrons from damaging you by keeping them under control.

Improved fitness

Co-Q was put to the test in a trial by scientists at the Free University in Brussels. They tested sedentary young men, supplementing with 60mg of Co-Q daily, and found improved endurance and heart strength after just four weeks. In other words, they were fitter – without exercising! While it goes without saying that we encourage everyone to keep fit by taking regular exercise, the evidence suggests that Co-Q supplementation maintains a level of fitness in sedentary people without exercise and improves fitness in people who do exercise. Also, adding Co-Q to any sports programme would be a good idea because aerobic exercise accelerates free radical production.

Better circulation

The well-documented strengthening effect of Co-Q on the heart muscle improves circulation, and therefore the supply of oxygen to all tissues. This increase in tissue oxygenation is another way that Co-Q can boost your energy level.

Co-Q has many other benefits too – boosting your immune system, helping to heal duodenal ulcers, reducing the side effects of cancer chemotherapy, alleviating histamine-related allergies and asthma, reducing high blood pressure and extending your life-span. It is truly a nutrient for the 21st century.

Where to Find It

Co-Q can be found in many foods, but not always in the form that we can make most use of. There are also many different types of Co-Q, ranging from Co-Q1 up to Co-Q10. Yeast, for example, contains Co-Q6 and Co-Q7. Only Co-Q10 is found in human tissues. It is this form of Co-Q that is effective in the ways described here and only this form should be supplemented. However, we can utilise 'lower' forms of dietary Co-Q and convert them into Co-Q10. This conversion process, which occurs in the liver, allows us to make use of the Co-Q found in almost all foods.

Some foods contain relatively more Co-Q10 than others, and it is probably these foods that are our best dietary sources of Co-Q. These include all meat and fish (especially mackerel, salmon and sardines), eggs, spinach, broccoli, alfalfa, potatoes, soya beans and soya oil, wheat (especially wheatgerm), rice bran, buckwheat, millet, and most beans, nuts and seeds.

Co-Q10 is also available in supplement form, and taking in extra in this way can really make your energy levels soar.

How and When to Take It and How Much

Levels of Co-Q10 present in the body decline with age, so it is especially recommended for those over 50. Exactly why and to what extent the conversion of lower forms of Co-Q into the active Co-Q10 is impaired is not known, but for people in this age group Co-Q10 is effectively an essential nutrient, and the

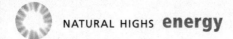
body needs to be given a supply of it, through either diet or supplements. The rest of us can also benefit from more Co-Q10 as an energy supplement. The best daily dosage is between 30 and 90mg a day, and 50mg is often recommended. It is best absorbed in an oil-soluble form.

Any Precautions?

No studies have reported toxicity of Co-Q even at extremely high doses taken over many years. There is no reason to assume that continued supplementation with Co-Q, as is advised for many vitamins, should have anything but extremely positive results.

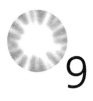

9

Dance to the Music

THERE ARE FEW THINGS that are as good at lifting the blues, boosting energy levels and rousing the spirit as bopping to a good beat. Music alone can be a great energiser. When your brain is stimulated, it produces beta waves, a certain pattern of activity that means you are alert and awake. By studying different kinds of music and their effects on the brain, we now know that listening to certain types of music, especially when dancing, can give you an immediate natural high.

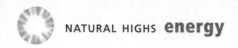

Why It's Good

Music promotes endorphins

Endorphins are the brain's own natural highs, released when you are happy, excited or having sex. Many drugs, from opium to cocaine, produce their euphoric effects by mimicking endorphins. And when scientists at the Addiction Research Center in Stanford, California, had people listen to various kinds of music, almost half the listeners reported feelings of euphoria, one of the signs of endorphins at work. To test this theory, the scientists injected listeners with naloxone, which blocks the brain's endorphin receptors. As a result, the listeners experienced far less euphoria, proving that music does boost endorphins.

Dancing gets you high

Both dancing and exercise, even without music, also promote endorphins in the brain, resulting in the well-known 'runner's high'. Research has proven that people who don't exercise are much more likely to suffer from low moods and depression than those who do. So pick up your running shoes, or even better, your dancing shoes. That's why, all throughout humanity's history there's been one sort of 'rave' after another. Music, coupled with dancing, is one of the best natural highs of them all.

What's the Best Music?

At one level, the best music is whatever you like. However, some of the music that gets the most beta waves going is made by brass bands and bagpipes! Certain rhythms have the same effect. No doubt that is why these types of music have been historically used when going into battle.

For the daily battles we all have to contend with these days, you might like to make your own CD or tape of stimulating music. Our favourites are listed on www.naturallyhigh.co.uk. This list includes all sorts of different kinds of music, from classical to contemporary, and notes the general effects of the music. With today's technology, it's getting easier to make your own selection of energy music to give you a lift whenever you need it.

Where to go Dancing

When was the last time you went dancing, or danced around your living room in gay abandon? We recommend dancing or moving to music almost every day, whether in that exercise class, at a party or concert, or by yourself at home. Instead of having a coffee, crank up the volume on your favourite track and lose yourself in the sound.

Gabrielle Roth, author of *Sweat Your Prayers*, says this about dancing: 'Energy moves in waves. Waves move in patterns. Patterns move in rhythms. A human being is just that, energy, waves, patterns, rhythms. Nothing more. Nothing less. A dance.' Music and dancing have the power to release feelings, inspire creativity and touch your soul. Roth invented Five Rhythms Dancing to do just that. At these wonderful evening 'classes', you can dance your socks off to a magical selection of music that takes you through on a journey, evoking all sorts of feelings, and leaving you in an undeniable state of natural ecstasy. Gabrielle Roth's classes are available throughout Britain. Just search for 'Five Rhythms' on the Web. Or take up any other form of dancing that appeals to you – from salsa to tango.

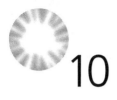

10

Energy Expenders – Eliminate Them

THERE ARE TWO SIDES to the energy equation: generating it, and consuming it. We consume the energy available to us in many ways, and sometimes, if we fail to generate enough, get 'burnt out'. Stimulants, from caffeine to cocaine, can be thought of as energy consumers. The 'high' is literally energy leaving the system, like the wave that breaks and seems, for a few seconds, to be full of energy. A few seconds later there is no wave at all. The energy is gone.

How You Deplete Your Energy

One of the models we have found most useful for understanding how and why we do things that deplete our energy is described by the world-renowned philosopher Oscar Ichazo, founder of the Arica School, a school of knowledge. In an article on drug abuse he says:

> Drugs (all of them) can be characterised as 'energy consumers', consuming energy at a rate much greater than our natural ability to replace it. As drugs burn all our accumulated vitality in short periods of time, the brief exaltation is inevitably followed by depletion of vital energy, felt as the 'down', the depressant effect of drugs. Nothing can replace a natural, clean body capable of producing natural and clean vital energy.

Ichazo rates the drugs most damaging to our vital energy in this order: alcohol, heroin and opiates, tobacco, cocaine, barbiturates, antidepressants, amphetamines, marijuana and caffeine.

The Doors of Compensation

Ichazo's model, called the Doors of Compensation, describes the nine different ways we dissipate energy – stimulants and drugs are just two of these. Compensating in one way or another is completely natural and can be seen as the way we keep ourselves psychologically in balance.

Think of your consciousness – your psyche – as a container. When we react to situations with emotional tension, when things don't go the way we expected, when we experience stress in one form or another, the pressure in our psyche increases. To release the pressure we use one or more of these doors of compensation. That's why, after a stressful week at work, people go out boozing on Friday night to let off steam, or take it out on the family by being bad-tempered, or stuff themselves full of food. Each of these is a way to dissipate energy and reduce the psyche's tension.

Understanding how we use these Doors of Compensation helps to identify sources of stress and allows us to develop healthier ways of staying in balance to support a productive and happy life. This process of self-discovery is the purpose of an extremely useful one-day training course called The Doors of Compensation. Details are in the Resources section on page 147.

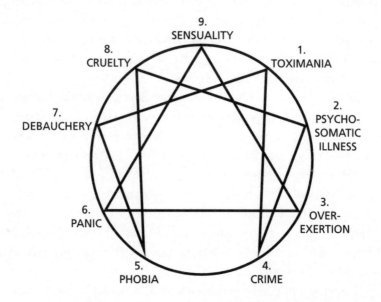

The Doors of Compensation Enneagram

The Doors of Compensation include:

1. **Toximania** – the use of substances including cigarettes, alcohol and caffeine

2. **Psychosomatic illness** – preoccupation with issues concerning mental and physical health and actual illness

3. **Over-exertion** – might manifest as workaholism or excessive activity

4. **Crime** – ways of getting even because you didn't feel you got a fair deal

5. **Phobia** – persistent, irrational fears as well as social aversions

6. **Panic** – fear and alarm, including fright about the future

7. **Debauchery (excess)** – which could manifest as excessive intake, for example of food

8. **Cruelty** – lack of compassion, as when being rude, using abusive language and cruel behaviour, and

9. **Sensuality** – which refers to pleasurable stimulation of any of the senses.

Each Door of Compensation relates to a particular area of life experience where a specific psychological imbalance occurs. For example, when we have stress in our work, we fear a loss of our productivity, and this makes us panic. So, having the objectivity to notice which 'doors' are attractive to you to use also shows the aspects of your life where your perceptions are generating internal pressure.

While we all use these ways of compensating at different times during every day, the degree to which we use them is also significant. The first degree of use is just occasionally, for temporary satisfaction. For example, you may have a couple of drinks after a stressful week on the odd occasion. The next degree is when you drink every day and you are anaesthetised by it. The third degree is when you habitually drink until you're drunk, which is debilitating. By this stage you are addicted to some degree, which represents a continual dissipation of energy.

11

Exercise for Energy

WE ALL KNOW IT: exercise is good for you. A bit of regular exertion and activity will ultimately result in you feeling more 'on your toes' more of the time. But the tricky thing is getting started. If you lack the energy even to take that first jog, swim or aerobics workout, the best course of action is simply to start. Soon you'll find you have a healthy portion of energy left over, to keep you fired up and invigorated throughout the day.

Exercise is an essential part of the energy equation, not only because it oxygenates the body – and energy can't be made

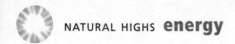

without oxygen – but also because movement itself gives you energy. We human beings are designed to keep moderately fit and, if you don't, you'll end up fatigued. Here's why.

Why It's Good

Makes you high and happy

Remember 'runner's high'? This happens when exercise promotes the release of endorphins, the brain's own feelgood factor. But there's more to it than that. Thanks to the research of Dr Dennis Lobstein from the University of New Mexico, we now know that people who exercise regularly are much less likely to be depressed or anxious than those who don't. He compared joggers to people living more sedentary lives and found that, quite apart from the high that the joggers experienced during exercise, they were consistently more emotionally stable, and less depressed or neurotic.[9]

Gives you energy and increases metabolism

Exercise also generates energy. The more you exercise, the less tired you feel. One of the main reasons for this is that it increases your metabolic rate, effectively turning up the 'fire' so you make more energy for both body and mind.

According to Professor McArdle, exercise physiologist at City University of New York, 'Most people can generate metabolic rates that are eight to ten times above their resting value during sustained cycling, running or swimming. Complementing this increased metabolic rate is the observation that vigorous exercise will raise metabolic rate for up to fifteen hours after exercise.'[10]

Stabilises your blood sugar

We are designed for exercise and, without it, the body losses its ability to balance blood sugar. The more you exercise, the more you lower your risk of blood sugar problems and diabetes.

Exercise is especially important in middle age because as we age, we are less likely to be able to maintain an even blood sugar level. A study of 87,000 women aged between 34 and 59 showed that those taking vigorous exercise at least once a week reduced their risk of diabetes by a third, compared to those who didn't work out.[11] While insulin levels don't necessarily decline with age, sensitivity to insulin does – a phenomenon known as insulin resistance. Physical activity in middle age and the elderly improves insulin sensitivity and therefore helps to stabilise blood sugar levels and weight.[12] Improved insulin resistance means more stable and consistent energy levels.

Burns fat and makes muscle

The best kind of exercise also helps to burn fat efficiently and make muscle. This includes brisk walking, jogging, cycling, swimming, aerobic dance, stepping, cross-country skiing, circuit training or any aerobic exercise that is steady, continuous and of a certain intensity. Since muscle cells consume more calories and make more energy than fat cells, the more lean muscle and less fat you have, the more energy your body produces and the more you are able to burn off excess calories.

How Often and How Much?

To get all these benefits, you need to exercise regularly. If you choose the right aerobic exercise that gets you puffing, you only need 2 hours exercise a week to make a difference. That's 15 minutes a day, or 21 minutes of exercise 5 days a week, giving yourself 2 days off. Alternatively, you may choose to 'double up' and exercise 3 times a week for 35 minutes at a time. It's pretty easy to manage.

What and Where?

You want aerobic exercise that builds stamina, exercise that builds muscle, and exercise that keeps you supple. Jogging and brisk walking help build up your stamina. Swimming is excellent for both stamina and strength. Psychocalisthenics (see page 103) is good for all three and can be done at home. Yoga is great for suppleness. If you join your local gym or health club you could also include a session on machines to improve your muscle tone, plus a couple of exercise or yoga classes a week.

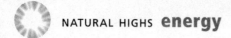

So every week, you could do something outside such as go running, do something at home, like light weight sessions, and go to the local gym for an exercise class or two.

Any Precautions?

Choose a form of exercise that you like. If you can, do it with a friend and build up your exercise intensity gradually. The more unfit you are to start with, the more benefit you'll get from seemingly small amounts of exercise. Rome wasn't built in a day. If you get bored, change your form of exercise.

12

Foods for Energy

W E ARE SOLAR-POWERED: the energy we need from food comes from the Sun. Plants use the Sun's energy to combine water from the soil and carbon dioxide from the air to make carbohydrate. We eat the plant, break the carbohydrate down into glucose and release the Sun's energy contained within it.

The foods to eat for high energy are the foods that can be most efficiently turned into energy in the body. In the early days of nutritional science it was thought that sugar – effectively pure body fuel – would be the best energy food. However, we now know that a high-sugar diet lacks the micronutrients

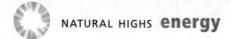

needed to turn it efficiently into energy; and because it is so 'high octane', it disrupts blood sugar levels.

Today the search is on for 'miles per gallon' – discovering which foods allow the human body to function efficiently, with stable blood sugar control, and an ideal all-round supply of the many nutrients involved in maintaining a consistent energy. Not surprisingly, this line of enquiry has led us right back to the very foods we evolved to eat – unrefined, organic, nutrient-rich wholefoods with an emphasis on lots of vegetables and fruit. And 'slow-releasing' carbohydrates are the real stars here.

Why They're Good

Carbohydrates such as wholewheat pasta or brown rice release their energy-giving carbohydrate slowly, giving you a consistent and sustained energy. These are the best foods:

Oats and oat flakes are the best cereal of all, better than wheat and cornflakes. In the winter you can make porridge; in the summer just have oat flakes – but not the sweetened variety.

You can sweeten them with fresh fruit. Oat cakes are great as a snack.

Whole rye bread is the best bread of all. Wholegrain bread is more 'slow-releasing' than refined, and rye bread is more slow-releasing than wheat bread. You can buy 100 per cent whole rye loaves in most supermarkets. Also great are German and Scandinavian-style breads such as pumpernickel and volken-brot. These both taste great and give you sustained energy.

Wholewheat pasta is much more slow-releasing than refined pasta. So too is buckwheat pasta or noodles, a staple food in Japanese diets. These slow-releasing pastas are widely available in supermarkets and health food shops.

Brown basmati rice is one of the best slow-releasing carbohydrates. While brown is generally better than white, basmati rice has less of a fast-releasing sugar called amylopectin, found in other strains of rice. It tastes just as good, if not better.

Beans and lentils are the best energy foods of all. This includes

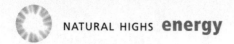

all beans including baked beans, kidney beans, black-eyed beans, tofu and other soya products, all lentils, quinoa, chickpeas and the chickpea paste hummus. These are a staple food for half the world. Also great are nuts and seeds.

Apples, pears and berries are the best fruit of all for energy. Having said that, all fruit can be classified as high-energy foods. It's just that apples, pears and berries are especially slow-releasing and therefore tend to give you more sustained energy.

All vegetables are 'whole foods' and that's what you want to be eating – something you could have pulled out of the ground or plucked from a bush.

If half your diet consists of these whole foods, you are on the right track for natural energy. The other side of the coin is to avoid refined sugars, including honey, as well as refined carbohydrates such as white bread, biscuits, cakes, white rice and other processed foods.

When and How?

When you eat and what you eat it with are as important as what you eat. The most important meal of the day is breakfast. Many people skip breakfast or have a cup of coffee and a piece of toast. What you eat for breakfast determines how you feel for the rest of the morning. So have a decent breakfast.

A diet high in fruit and vegetables, while good for your energy and health, is simply not as filling as our traditional high-fat, high-protein diet. This means you may need to snack on fruit mid-morning and mid-afternoon. Studies comparing the effects of eating little and often, compared to a couple of large meals a day, consistently show better health for those who 'graze' rather than gorge.

If your day is stressful, have a light lunch that requires little digestion, but most importantly, get out of the office, put your feet up and stop thinking about work – even if for only 15 minutes. You need at least two hours to complete the first stage of digesting a meal, so dinner should never be later than two hours before the time you go to sleep.

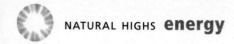
Contrary to popular myth, combining protein-rich foods such as fish, chicken or tofu with carbohydrate-rich foods such as rice, pasta or potatoes helps to further stabilise your blood sugar level and to promote a high, consistent energy level. So, salmon and brown basmati rice, or vegetable and tofu stir-fry with wholewheat pasta, are high-energy meals.

13

Ginseng – King of All Tonics

WHEN WE THINK of pick-me-ups, we tend to see them as good for getting us up and running, but not for keeping us that way. A less fleeting restorative might sound too good to be true, but it's not. Ginseng is out there waiting to prove to us that there really is something that can not only invigorate you when you're flagging, but also provide you with enough oomph to put new heart into long-term pursuits.

For some 5,000 years, ginseng has been revered in China as a general tonic that increases your energy and sense of well-being. Such was the status of this shrub, which is native to the

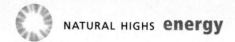
woodlands of Northern China, Korea and Siberia, that warlords of the region are said to have battled over the ground where it grew.

There are actually several related herbs commonly called ginseng, but the two most commonly used are Korean ginseng (*Panax ginseng*) and Siberian ginseng (*Eleutherococcus senticosus*). The latter, while related, is technically not a ginseng, though its functions are very similar.

Russians have known about the benefits of ginseng for decades, using it to improve athletic performance and to help cosmonauts remain alert and energetic despite the considerable physical and mental stresses of life in space. Taking ginseng regularly improves your endurance and capacity to handle stress and heavy workloads, with less strain on your mind and body.

Why It's Good

Ginseng is an energy tonic. As such, it is not generally regarded as having specific disease-fighting properties, but rather acts *with* the body to adjust and adapt to stressful conditions. Ancient

Chinese texts (the emperor Sh'eng Nung's *Materia Medica*) describe it as 'a tonic to the five viscera: quieting the spirits, establishing the soul, allaying fear, expelling evil affluvia, brightening the eyes, opening the heart, benefiting the understanding, invigorating the body and prolonging life'. Quite a review!

Ginseng is now one of the most researched of all herbs, and modern science is confirming what the Chinese have known for thousands of years. Most of this research has been conducted in Russia, and has confirmed that ginseng improves our capacity to withstand physical stress, increases our mental alertness and work output, and improves our quality of work and even athletic performance.

Better stress tolerance

A key role of tonics like ginseng is helping the body adapt to stresses of all kinds – mental, physical and environmental – by supporting the adrenal glands, your stress responders. Ginseng helps normalise the way the body responds to stress, calming things down if you're overstressed, and energising you if you need a boost. It also strengthens the adrenal glands themselves,

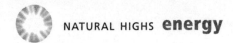

which is especially important to those suffering from chronic stress. And as stress affects so many of us today, adaptogenic tonics like ginseng are more helpful than ever.

Better concentration, performance and mood

The stress-protective and performance-enhancing effects of taking ginseng have been confirmed in many trials. In one study with Russian telegraph workers, subjects were asked to transmit the same piece of text rapidly and continuously for five minutes. While all the participants transmitted similar numbers of characters in the allotted time, those who were taking ginseng made significantly fewer errors.[13] Two reviews of dozens of experiments involving over 2,000 people taking ginseng for up to three months confirmed its ability to improve mood and intellectual performance, with almost no side effects.[14]

More energy

As well as protecting from stress, Siberian ginseng increases the supply of oxygen to cells, thereby boosting endurance, alertness and visual-motor coordination. It can also normalise blood pressure and blood sugar levels – vital for consistent energy levels without the highs and lows brought on by other stimulants, sugars and refined carbohydrates. Ginseng has the rare ability to boost both immediate and long-term energy.

Where to Find It

While ginseng is now extremely rare in the wild, it's farmed in Korea, China, Russia and Japan. The dried powdered roots of Siberian and Korean ginsengs are available in health food shops as teas, tinctures, tablets and capsules. American ginseng has calming rather than stimulating properties, so if it's energy your after, go for the Asian varieties.

How and When to Take It and How Much

When you're overworked, stressed or exhausted, ginseng is an ideal antidote. It can be used safely to help you through short periods of excessively difficult periods (bereavement, exams, moving house, divorce, redundancy, etc.), or as a general tonic to help you cope with the stresses of daily life.

The recommended dose of Korean ginseng is 100mg once or twice daily of a dried root extract containing 4 to 7 per cent of the active ingredients, called ginsenosides. As Korean ginseng is generally considered quite 'yang' (a stimulating and strengthening herb), Siberian ginseng is recommended for women (see precautions, opposite).

Take 200mg of dried root and extract of Siberian ginseng (containing at least 1 per cent eleutherosides) once or twice daily. If using a tincture, take 5ml twice daily in a little water. The tincture should be around five parts alcohol to one part ginseng.

Chinese tradition recommends taking ginseng as part of a two-month restorative programme, using this time to gather and store energy by eating well, resting, relaxing, exercising, avoiding stress, and completely eliminating drugs and alcohol. Combined with regular ginseng intake, such a programme can really give you back your get up and go.

Any Precautions?

Side effects at the doses above are very rare, though overuse of ginseng can cause overstimulation, leading to insomnia, irritability and anxiety. Unconfirmed reports of excessive doses raising blood pressure and increasing heart rate have been largely discredited, though Korean ginseng should be avoided in cases of high blood pressure unless advised by a qualified medical practitioner. Korean ginseng is generally recommended only for men, as it can cause menstrual irregularities, such as prolonged menstrual bleeding, and breast tenderness in some women. All ginsengs, including Siberian, should be taken for no more than three months at a time, and after that, used as a tonic when needed.

Some recommend ginseng during pregnancy, and others warn against it. As with all herbs, if you're pregnant, consult a qualified herbal practitioner before you use it.

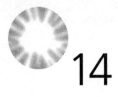

14

Green Tea – Good Health in a Cup

GREEN TEA (*CAMELLIA SINESIS*) is made from the dried leaves of an evergreen shrub native to Asia. Chinese legend has it that the Emperor Sh'eng Nung took the first sip of tea in about 2737 BC, when some leaves accidentally blew into his cooking pot. Since then, tea has become the most popular beverage in the world, after water. Archaeological evidence indicates that tea leaves steeped in boiling water were consumed by *Homo erectus pekinensis* more than 500,000 years ago.

Contrary to popular belief, green tea is actually exactly the same plant as normal, black tea, and it does contain caffeine, although not as much as black tea. The difference between the two is that black tea has been fermented, while green tea is made from only the leaf bud and the top two leaves, which are lightly steamed to preserve them without destroying the beneficial compounds.

For centuries, the Chinese have extolled the health benefits of green tea, and now scientific research is endorsing their claims. Rich in antioxidants, flavonoids, glycosides, vitamins and minerals, green tea is much more than a refreshing drink. According to Diana Rosen, author of *Green Tea: Good Health in Your Cup*, 'Tea is a retreat in a cup. Give it time and it can give you greater clarity of thought and a clearer sense of purpose. You can get lost in tea. You can find yourself in tea. In fact, tea can change your life.'[15]

While we can't guarantee it'll change your life, green tea is a great natural stimulant with many other health benefits too.

Why It's Good

Green tea contains certain important health-giving compounds – especially polyphenols – that are potent antioxidants with

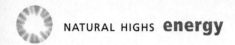

cancer-protective and anti-ageing effects. Black tea also contains these compounds, but with proportionately more caffeine along with them.

Mild stimulant

Considering the many other health benefits of green tea, in moderation (meaning no more than around four cups a day) it's a useful natural stimulant. This stimulant effect is partly due to the caffeine content, though green tea contains only 20 to 30mg of caffeine per cup, as compared to 50mg in a regular cup of tea and 100mg in a regular cup of coffee. As a result it is less stimulating, and for some it's even relaxing. Green tea also contains theanine, a mild stimulant which reduces the excitatory effect of caffeine. In fact, Asian monks have traditionally used it to help keep them awake, though still calm, during meditation practice.

Less stress

This combination of stimulation and relaxation may be the key to green tea's ability to improve your stress tolerance. It's an ideal alternative to regular black tea and coffee, which disrupt blood sugar balance, rob the body of nutrients and can result in dependency, all adding to the stress on your mind and body instead of lowering it.

Stronger immunity

The beneficial compounds in green tea boost immunity and have proven anti-cancer properties even more powerful than vitamins C and E. Some believe that green tea consumption – three cups a day on average – is the reason for the relatively low rate of cancer in Japan. These compounds, especially flavonoids and glycosides, protect the body from damage caused by oxidants, and thereby support the immune system and can slow down the ageing process.

On top of all this, green tea has been shown to lower cholesterol and blood pressure, increase HDL – the so-called 'good' cholesterol – as well as thin the blood, reduce the risk of heart attack and stroke, prevent dental caries and aid weight loss by encouraging the body to burn fat. Maybe it *can* change your life!

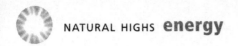

Where to Find It

Green tea is becoming more widely available in the UK. Major tea manufacturers are now selling it, though specialist brands, which are often hand-processed and tend to be better quality, are available in speciality and health food stores. Japanese green teas are particularly good. Also available, if you're after a therapeutically high intake of antioxidants, are tinctures of green tea extract or capsules of powdered green tea.

How and When to Take It and How Much

You can drink two to six cups of green tea daily, steeped to taste, though be aware that green tea is generally steeped for only two minutes or so, and longer than this makes the tea more bitter. We recommend taking Diana Rosen's advice to try and relax over your cup of green tea. 'Tea requires time,' she says. 'If you give enough quality time to tea, it will reward you with more than you ever imagined. It's just you, your thoughts, and the magic of your bowl of tea.'

With the infinitely less romantic but more potent green tea capsules, take 300 to 400mg daily and choose ones standardised to contain at least 50 per cent polyphenols.

Any Precautions?

If you drink more than eight cups of green tea a day, you'll be taking in a lot of caffeine. This can cause typical caffeine effects such as nervousness, insomnia and restlessness in some individuals. Because of the potential of green tea to thin the blood, those taking aspirin or anticoagulant substances on a daily basis should be aware of potential additive effects and consult their doctor before they drink green tea or take green tea supplements regularly.

15

Licorice – the Natural Pick-me-up

ARE YOU PERPETUALLY LOW on energy? Is pain wearing you down, or a cough robbing you of enough oxygen to stay energised? It sounds as if you might not find a sweeter antidote than the goodness contained in a quick fix of licorice.

Licorice (*Glycyrrhiza glabra*) is a purple and white flowering plant native to the Mediterranean and central and southwest Asia, and is now grown in many parts of the world. While you may think of it as the popular sweet, licorice root is one of the most ancient herbal medicines known. It's been appreciated for its medicinal qualities for over 3,000 years in Chinese traditional medicine, and has even been found in the tombs of ancient Egyptian pharaohs. It was, and still is, used as a rejuvenating tonic and as an expectorant, useful in treating flu, colds, respiratory disorders and bronchitis, and is also helpful in the treatment of gastric and duodenal ulcers.

Why It's Good

The medicinal benefits of licorice root have been studied extensively, and its use in traditional medicine is well documented. Medical researchers have isolated several active substances in licorice root, including glycosides, flavonoids, asparagine, isoflavonoids, chalcones, coumarins, and oestrogenic substances, which lend the herb oestrogen-like effects. It's also rich in nutrients including vitamin E, B-complex, phosphorous, biotin, niacin, pantothenic acid, lecithin, manganese, iodine, chromium and zinc.

All in all, licorice is a very impressive herb, and its qualities are well supported by medical research and clinical data. The key benefit of licorice root for energy is that is provides

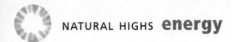

support for the adrenal glands (your stress responders), helping with mild adrenal insufficiency and low blood sugar.

Better stress response

Traditional Chinese medicine uses licorice to replenish your *chi*, or vital energy, and modern science is now showing us how. Chronic stress can lead to the adrenals becoming exhausted – a precursor to chronic fatigue – and licorice can give you the lift you need. While we generally talk about the adrenal hormone cortisol as a bad thing (which it is if it's too high for too long), it is essential for our short-term response to stress. Licorice elevates cortisol by preventing its breakdown, so if you take licorice, the cortisol you make lasts longer.[16] This is bad news if you've got high cortisol already, for example in the alarm stage of stress, but good news if chronic or long-term stress has exhausted your adrenals to the point where they can no longer make enough cortisol for you to deal with what the world throws at you. (See when to take it, page 88.)

Less pain and inflammation

If pain and inflammation are sapping your energy, licorice has another helpful effect. Because cortisol decreases pain and inflammation, and licorice raises it, licorice can act as a herbal anti-inflammatory and anti-arthritic agent, and is recognised as a time-honoured remedy for arthritis due to its anti-inflammatory properties. The anti-ulcer benefits of licorice are also widely recognised, though generally the deglycyrrhizinated form is recommended, which can't help your energy levels.

Raises blood pressure

If you have low blood pressure, which often accompanies chronic fatigue, licorice comes to the rescue again. Low blood pressure starves the brain of oxygen and nutrients, so keeping your blood flowing is vital to feeling alert and energetic. Licorice can raise blood pressure by causing more sodium to be retained. Be careful, though: this can go too far and lead to *high* blood pressure in susceptible individuals (see precautions, page 90).

Breathe easier

Oxygen is our most important 'nutrient' for energy production. Every cell is completely dependent on it, and respiratory problems such as colds and flu certainly aren't going to help. Licorice's expectorant qualities are well recognised, so it's a key ingredient in nearly any cough remedy you care to look at. By keeping those airways clear, your breathing and therefore oxygen supply to the brain and body will be unobstructed.

How and When to Take It and How Much

As a tincture, take 5ml in a little water three times a day. Or take one to three 500mg licorice root capsules twice a day. Licorice tea is made by simmering half a teaspoon of dried powder in 300ml of water for 10 minutes before straining, and can be drunk twice a day. In general, take licorice in the morning and midday rather than in the evening, as cortisol levels should be naturally falling at this time.

To know if you should take licorice, and at what specific times in the day, a saliva-based Adrenal Stress Index test (available through nutrition consultants) can show you what your cortisol levels are doing throughout the day, when you should boost them, and when you needn't.

Note: Deglycyrrhizinated licorice, recommended to those who want the anti-ulcer activity of licorice without risking raising their blood pressure, does *not* have the hormone-like action of licorice that can benefit your energy levels and stress response.

Where to Find It

Licorice is sold almost everywhere as a popular sweet, though many such products don't actually contain any real licorice, and if they do, the level is very low. Health food stores and herbalists sell powdered licorice from which you can make tea, or whole licorice roots to chew (it's nicer than it sounds). Licorice tea bags are widely available, as are licorice tinctures and capsules.

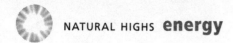

Any Precautions?

The active component in licorice, glycyrrhizin, can cause fluid retention and raise blood pressure, so avoid long-term use of large doses without professional supervision. Clearly, if you already have raised blood pressure or cortisol levels, or are on corticoid (steroid) or diuretic medications, licorice is not recommended. There are no reports of interactions with other medications, though licorice is not recommended during pregnancy, breastfeeding or for children under five because of its hormonal effects.

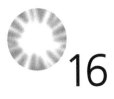

16

Meditation – Free Your Mind

MEDITATION – ISN'T IT all about 'peacing out'? Surely it can't give you the immediate fizz and sparkle you crave? But it can: feeling altogether more sharp and keen is such a fundamental by-product of meditation that it can't even be labelled a secondary effect. If you're hankering after a steady flow of verve and liveliness, you'll be pleasantly surprised by the energising upshot of such a peaceful practice.

Meditation is an ancient, established route to feeling naturally high, energised and happy. It works by expanding your awareness beyond the mind and body, and promoting a feeling

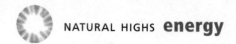

of calm and contentment. Far from being an activity confined to monks and latter-day hippies, meditation is a thoroughly practical tool for managing the stresses of daily living.

Why It's Good

Meditation is the ultimate antidote to the effects of stress on every level. Physically, it reduces heart rate and blood pressure, slows the rate of breathing and stabilises brain-wave patterns. It also improves the body's responsiveness to stressful events and aids quicker recovery. In addition, it has been shown to prevent the depression of the body's immune responses that occurs with stress.

Clarity and peace of mind

The benefits of meditation on mental and emotional health are far-reaching. There's no doubt that meditation helps dissolve anxiety and promotes clarity and calm. In fact, people who practise meditation on a regular basis have been found to be less anxious than those who don't, and research has found that medi-tators have lower levels of the stress hormone cortisol.

This is no small thing. Although we cannot change what happens to us from day to day, we can change the way we *respond* to stressful situations. Regular meditation helps us become less reactive to the normal stresses and strains of life.

Energise the mind

Most meditation techniques involve focusing on one object as a way to calm the mind. This could be a mantra such as 'Om', the flame of a candle, or the breath. Research at the Heffter Institute in California (see www.heffter.org) on the effects of focusing on the breath suggests that this helps bring the brain into balance. As the mind becomes quieter, your powers of concentration and mental agility improve. You are more able to focus your energy on the task at hand, instead of dissipating energy by trying to 'multi-task' without doing any individual task completely.

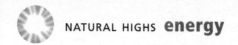

How Often and How Much?

Meditation is much like physical exercise: it is more beneficial to meditate for 10 minutes every day than to meditate for an hour once a week. Daily practice – even if it's only for a few minutes – will quickly get your mind into the habit of meditating.

When you first start meditating, give yourself a realistic time-frame. Start with at least 10 minutes every day. Gradually increase the time to 15 minutes, and so on. There is no time limit to meditation: you need to see what feels best for you.

How to do It – the Basics

Try and find a quiet place. It can help to sit in darkness, as this helps the mind to settle down. You may find it easiest to meditate first thing in the morning or last thing at night, when the mind tends to be relatively quiet.

Posture

The foundation for meditation is good posture. If your body feels at ease, then the mind finds it easier to relax. Your spine should be straight but not rigid. If you sit on the floor, sit in a comfortable cross-legged posture. It often helps to sit on a cushion as this tips the pelvis forward and naturally supports the spine. Some people like to sit with their back against a wall for support.

If you prefer to sit on a chair, then sitting forward in your seat helps straighten the spine. Place your feet flat on the floor – if your feet don't reach the floor, place a cushion underneath them.

It's vital to feel comfortable: meditation is about relaxation, after all.

Breathing

Once you've found a comfortable posture, focus your attention on your breath and begin Diakath Breathing (see page 28).

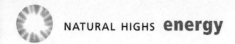

Focus your mind

Keep your mind gently focused on your breath as it comes in and goes out. Bring your awareness to the place from where your breath arises. Good meditation doesn't have to mean that you are completely free of thoughts. If your mind does wander, simply become aware that your focus has shifted to your thoughts and bring it back to your breath.

Where to Find Details

Approaches and courses abound. For details of courses in your area, see the Reources section on page 147.

17

The Present – Live in It

L IFE IS A STRING of present moments. Most of us spend most of these moments thinking about the past or worrying about the future. This is exhausting and unproductive. Psychologists tell us that we have at least 6,000 thoughts in a day, and most of them are repeats! Our minds spend enormous amounts of energy going over things in the past, and anticipating things in the future, rather than being in the present. Yet being in the present is a natural energy high.

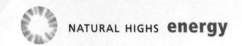

How to do It

Finish unfinished business

The single greatest cause of feeling overwhelmed is having unfinished business. Make a list of everything that is unfinished in your life. Then, one by one, finish each item. It may be a practical task, or something you need to say to someone, or a past relationship that needs completing.

Do it completely

When you have something to do, do it completely. Don't half do it, then start doing something else.

Make an appointment to deal with it later

If, during the day, something upsets you, or you realise there is something else you need to do, make an appointment to deal with it later, by writing it down. Either allocate a time to it in your diary if it is a job for you to do, or, if perhaps someone upset you, put it on your 'unfinished business' page and review the incident, and what action, if any, you wish to take, at the end of the day. If you don't do this, chances are you are going to go over and over the incident, or keep remembering the thing you have to do, again and again and again. Writing it down helps you keep doing. It's amazing how the mind lets go once you've made an appointment to deal with something later.

Throw away your 'to do' list

Endless 'to do' lists can drive you crazy. You wake up thinking about all the things you haven't done. Since the only time that exists is the present, decide what you are going to do today and do it. A list of four or five things you are going to do today is fine, but an endless list is a constant source of anxiety.

Learn how to manage your time effectively

If you always give yourself too much to do, start being realistic about what you can and can't do. Try doing this by allocating one 'catch-up' day a week for all those little jobs that get in the way of your more critical projects. Also, start your day by completing an important job first.

File according to time, not type

Instead of having piles of 'bills to pay', 'things to read', 'letters to write' and other endless visible reminders of things to do, file what you're going to do on the day you're going to do it. I (Patrick) have a filing system called a 'time existence' system. It looks like a portable 'squeeze box', with sections labelled 1 to 31 for the days of the month. You can buy these in stationers' shops. I file tasks in see-through plastic folders, with all the papers I need for that job, in the day I've allocated in my diary to do them. That way, I can forget about them until their time has come!

When a new job comes my way, or when I open the post in the morning, I either complete the assignment there and then – and it's done. Or I allocate a time or day to do it, file it in my 'squeeze box' and forget about it. Or I realise I will never do this thing, and bin it. No more piles of papers reminding me of all the things I have to do, half of which I never will.

Develop a regular practice of techniques that keep you focused

Learn how to keep yourself in the present. Meditation, yoga, t'ai chi and breathing exercises such as Diakath Breathing (see page 28) all help you to stay in the present. A simple technique in meditation, when your mind drifts off, is to bring your focus back to the breath. The same applies in your daily life.

Another technique for keeping your awareness in the present is to include your body in your field of awareness. Practise this for five minutes and you will notice how your mind quietens down and how much more observant you become. When we are out of the present, with minds whizzing from past regrets to future fantasies, we forget we even have a body. By including your body in your field of awareness, you can bring yourself back to the present moment.

Another technique for developing focused attention and the ability to stay in the present is becoming aware of the silence behind all sound. Do this for a few minutes. Become aware of all the sounds around you. Become aware that all these sounds emerge from silence and dissolve back into silence. Practising

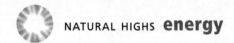

this for a few minutes every day, even perhaps when you go to buy you lunch at work, helps to quieten the mind and develop your ability to stay grounded in the present.

Give yourself some time to do nothing, and time to yourself

We all need time to do nothing. Give yourself at least a day, or two half days, where nothing is scheduled. Do whatever you want to do, including nothing. Also give yourself some time to yourself, at least a day a month.

Remember, 'The past is history, the future a mystery, all that exists is the present. It's a gift – that's why it's called "the present".'

18

Psychocalisthenics

Your energy levels don't just come from the food you eat. They're also dependent on the state of your body. Without exercise, the body loses muscle tone and it accumulates tension – and you feel tired. Exercise improves the circulation and oxygenates the blood, which is a natural high in itself. But there's another type of energy.

This is 'vital energy'. Masters from every tradition of self-transformation have learnt how to tap into it. In China it's called *chi*. In Japan it's called *ki*. In India it's called *prana*. T'ai chi and aikido are examples of exercises to increase your vital energy.

All of them give you extra energy and health benefits beyond those of regular exercise.

In essence, vital energy is produced by focusing attention in the body's centre of balance, three finger-widths below the navel. This energy centre is known in t'ai chi as the *tantien* and in the Arica system (see page 105) as Kath[sm]. Awareness of this point has the power to nourish us at a fundamental level. Vital energy increases our awareness of our whole body, allowing us to feel at peace with the world around us.

What It Is

Our all-time favourite vital energy exercise is Psychocalisthenics.[a] You can learn this in five hours, by watching a video or in a course, and do it in 15 minutes wherever you are. There are no gadgets required, just a precise sequence of exercises that leave you feeling fantastic. After doing Psychocalisthenics you feel energised and ready for action, yet calm and centre at the

[a] © 2002 Oscar Ichazo. Psychocalisthenics is a registered trademark of Oscar Ichazo. Used by permission.

same time. Each exercise is driven by the breath and, somehow, your body feels lighter, freer and thoroughly oxygenated after this simple routine.

Psychocalisthenics is the brainchild of Oscar Ichazo, whose work we first discussed in Chapter 5. Ichazo founded the Arica School in the 1960s for the understanding of the complete person. A practitioner of martial arts and yoga since 1939, he developed Psychocalisthenics as a daily routine of 23 exercises that can be done in less than 20 minutes. Psychocalisthenics is a complete contemporary exercise system which, at first glance, looks like a powerful kind of aerobic yoga. 'In the same way that we have an everyday need for food and nourishment we have to promote the circulation of our vital energy as an everyday business,' says Ichazo.

Why It's Good

So, while most exercise routines simply treat the body as a physical machine that needs to be worked to stay fit, Psychocalisthenics is designed to generate both physical fitness and vital energy by bringing mind and body into balance.

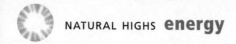

The key lies in the precise breathing pattern accompanying each physical exercise. 'Once we integrate our mind with our body across a controlled respiration, we can produce in ourselves an element of self-observation that is indispensable for acquiring understanding of our true nature,' says Ichazo. 'What Psychocalisthenics offers is a set of exercises that can become a serious foundation for a life of self-responsibility, clarity of mind and strength of spirit.'

Psychocalisthenics is a combination of movement, breathing exercises and Kath awareness. It is the Kath awareness that generates vital energy and this is what makes Psychocalisthenics unique – a perfect combination of East and West. Once you've learnt the routine you can do it at home, accompanied by the video or audiotape. It takes a day to learn and will leave you feeling blissful and energised.

How to Learn It

There are two ways to learn Psychocalisthenics.

1. **One-day Psychocalisthenics training**
   This is the fastest, most effective and enjoyable way of learning the exercises in a single day. These training courses are held frequently in different parts of the UK.

2. **Teach yourself with a self-tuition kit**
   You can teach yourself by ordering the self-tuition kit, which includes the book *Master Level Exercise, Psychocalisthenics* by Oscar Ichazo, a video, a wall chart and a music cassette.

See Resources, page 147, for further details.

19

Reishi – the Japanese Energy Secret

WE SAY SOMETHING 'mushroomed' when it sprang up suddenly and swiftly. So it's fitting that when we consume the reishi mushroom, our energy level gets a quick boost, and many other benefits – to our immune system, blood sugar level, heart and even lifespan – follow. The knock-on effects on all-round well-being from this ancient Asian fungus are prolific and plentiful.

The reishi mushroom (*Ganoderma lucidum*) is a wood-rotting fungus found on the sides of trees and stumps in many parts of the world, and is most used and researched in China and

Japan. Its glossy red cap and black stem may look unusual, but inside are phytochemicals that make it one of the most respected tonics in herbal medicine. In Asia it has been revered for 4,000 years, and used to help people adapt physically and mentally to the world. It strengthens and calms the nerves, improves memory, and prevents or delays senility.

Why It's Good

Reishi mushrooms are recommended as a general tonic for health, energy and longevity. Their use extends to almost every system of the body. Not only are they believed to heal physical ailments; they are also said to bring about a peaceful state of mind, sharpen your thinking, energise you when you're fatigued and even increase spiritual energy.

Energising

Reishi has been shown to be particularly beneficial as an energising tonic. In one clinical trial with 37 people reporting general weakness, insomnia, poor memory and tiredness, their symptoms were improved by 56 per cent in 4 to 6 weeks, after taking reishi. One way in which reishi might do this is via regulation of blood glucose, as it smoothes out the rises and falls in blood sugar common in those with poor energy control.

Calming

Among the many phytonutrients in reishi are compounds known as nucleosides, which are known muscle relaxants. Reishi has been shown to improve sleep quality, particularly deep sleep, and exert a calming effect on the central nervous system when tested in people.

Longer life

Most lifespan studies done today are with fruit flies. This species reproduces quickly and changes in its lifespan are easily observed. It is therefore of interest that when Chinese researchers put reishi mushroom extracts in their water, this prolonged the lifespans of both male and female fruit flies significantly, increasing their average and maximum lifespans by around 17 per cent.

Helps your heart

The heart-health effects of reishi mushrooms are truly remarkable. Reishi has been shown to reduce clot formation, lower blood pressure by up to 10 points, and can even lower cholesterol by up to 18 per cent!

Immune system boosting

Herbalists consider reishi an adaptogen, or natural regulator, suppressing the immune system if it is overactive and boosting it if it is underactive. Many health claims are made on the effect that reishi has on the immune system. These claims are based primarily on the presence of polysaccharides, antioxidants and the minerals potassium, magnesium, calcium and germanium in reishi extracts.

In addition to the above benefits, reishi has been shown to reduce the growth of tumours and the incidence of cancer in animal trials more than other known anti-cancer nutrients like beta-carotene and vitamin C. It can also improve vigour, appetite and recovery in cancer sufferers, reduce altitude sickness, benefit diabetics, and reduce inflammation. It's anti-microbial and a powerful antioxidant.

How and When to Take It and How Much

Reishi mushrooms are available dried and as powder, tinctures, tablets and capsules. Up to 9g of dried mushrooms in three equally divided dosages can be taken daily, though as a general health tonic, 2 to 4g daily is recommended in three equal portions, with meals. Teas can be made by boiling 3g dried mushrooms in a litre of water for two hours; drink this twice daily.

In combination products reishi is likely to appear as a more potent *extract*, and therefore effective doses can be much lower.

Where to Find It

Reishi products can be found in health food stores, herbalists and Chinese markets, often in combination products with other beneficial mushrooms like shiitake and maitake, or in natural energy formulas, together with other natural stimulants.

Any Precautions?

People with allergies to moulds or fungi should take care using reishi mushrooms, although allergic reactions to them are generally rare. In clinical studies, reishi mushrooms have been shown to be non-toxic in high doses, and severe side effects have not been observed. Mild side effects may include stomach upset, dry mouth, diarrhoea and skin rash, though these generally disappear after several days. Side effects can be alleviated by stopping use, or in the case of stomach upset and diarrhoea, taking the supplement with meals. Because reishi boosts the immune system, it is not advised for those receiving immuno-suppressive therapies.

20

Rhodiola – the Energy Elixir

THE WORD IS FINALLY OUT on a big energy secret that Siberians have known about for 3,000 years. It's a simple herb which keeps you feeling on top of the world, ready, alert and agile, and gives you the stamina and endurance to work and play hard. It's time we in the West wise up to the powerful properties of rhodiola.

Rhodiola grows in the Arctic regions of eastern Siberia and, according to Siberian folklore, it can help you live to 100 or more. For centuries, Chinese emperors in search of the elixer of life sent special expeditions to bring it back from the Arctic.

Why It's Good

Rhodiola doesn't just increase your energy levels; it has a range of other benefits, too. Although the claims that it will guarantee you that 100th-birthday telegram from Buckingham Palace may be overstated, it's not all folklore. Modern science is confirming that rhodiola can enhance your body's ability to adapt to both acute and chronic stress, thereby helping to eliminate fatigue, boost your physical and mental energy and increase immunity.

More energy

In Russia, rhodiola is an ingredient in energy drinks, and has also been used to improve athletic powers. In one study of 112 athletes, researchers found that the performance of 89 per cent of those supplementing rhodiola showed more rapid improvement than that of their teammates.[17]

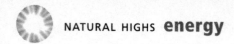

Less stress

In situations of stress, whether physical or mental, the energy boost provided by rhodiola can definitely give you that extra edge. In a study to assess its ability to help adapt to physical stress, 52 people aged 18 to 24 were put through a gruelling physical regime. Those supplementing rhodiola performed 12 per cent better than the controls, then 28 per cent better in a repeat of the test after they were all tired from the first one, indicating better physical stress tolerance and quicker recovery. In a similar trial investigating rhodiola's effect on mental stress, subjects given the herb during an extended period of intensive work experienced improved intellectual work capacity and made fewer errors. In a Russian placebo-controlled, double-blind study published in the journal *Phytomedicine*, researchers tested the physical and mental performance of 40 medical students during a stressful exam period. Those who took 50 mg of rhodiola twice daily for 20 days reported decreased mental fatigue and need for sleep, and scored 8 per cent better in their exams than those in the control group.[18]

Better concentration, better mood

The effects of rhodiola's energy high on the brain are perhaps the most interesting of all. Numerous studies have shown that it improves your concentration, especially when you're tired. In a proofreading test with 120 students aged 20 to 28, those taking rhodiola made 88 per cent fewer errors compared to those on the placebo! It also helps the brain make serotonin, the 'happy' neurotransmitter. In a study of 128 people suffering from depression, who were given 200mg of rhodiola, nearly two-thirds of the patients experienced a major reduction in or disappearance of their symptoms.

Stronger immunity

On top of all this, rhodiola boosts immunity and has proven anti-cancer properties, probably because it is exceptionally rich in antioxidant nutrients, especially flavonoids and proanthocyanidins. These protect the body from damage caused by oxidants, and thereby slow down the ageing process. They also help the body use other vital antioxidant nutrients such as vitamin C. Some researchers claim that proanthocyanidins (which

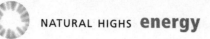

are also found in berries) are several times stronger than vitamins C and E. In any event, they are extremely good news as far as your immune system is concerned.

How and When to Take It and How Much

There's no question that rhodiola can give you an energy boost but, as with other herbs, make sure you are getting the real thing. There are many plant varieties of rhodiola, but the one that works best is called *Rhodiola rosea*. Of its many active ingredients, the key components are rosavin and salidroside. It is best to take rhodiola supplements that are standardised, and therefore guarantee that you are getting at least 2 per cent rosavin and 1 per cent salidroside. You need between 200mg and 300mg of such a standardised extract, taken one to three times per day with meals. Reduce this dose if you start to feel unmotivated due to too little stress.

Where to Find It

Rhodiola is now commonly available in health food shops as capsules or tablets, though be sure to get quality standardised products as suggested above.

Any Precautions?

At these levels, rhodiola is very safe, and has no reported side effects. It is considered even safer than Asian ginseng. However, excessive amounts have been reported to raise blood pressure, and it may therefore be unsuitable in higher doses for those with hypertension. Rhodiola is not recommended by some herbalists for pregnant women. If in doubt, consult your health practitioner.

21

Get Enough Sleep

THERE'S NOTHING QUITE LIKE that attentive and content state of mind we get from a good night's sleep. Sleep is essential 'nourishment' for both the body and the mind. It's like a blast of fresh air for mind and body. People who are stressed often have sleep-related problems, while a lack of sleep is itself a stress factor. If you want to be healthy and full of energy, you need to get enough good-quality sleep.

Why It's Good

Dreaming regenerates your mind

As far as the mind is concerned the most critical phases of sleep are bursts of REM (rapid eye movement) sleep, when dreams occur most frequently. These tend to start after an hour or so of sleep and last for about half an hour, occurring on average five to seven times a night. The longer you sleep the longer the REM phases last, which is why you need at least seven hours of sleep a night.

When deprived of REM sleep, you don't feel fully rested on waking and are more likely to get depressed. When people do get a chance to sleep, they have longer periods of REM sleep. All of this suggests that our minds need to have this time while we're asleep to process what's been happening in our lives. It is generally thought that dreams are important for mental and emotional health.

Promotes memory

During REM sleep the brain makes all sorts of neurotransmitters, from noradrenalin, which keeps you stimulated, to serotonin, which keeps you happy and improves your memory. Experiments by Dr Robert Stickgold at Harvard Medical School have found that we need sleep to remember what we've learnt during the day.[19] He found that the ability to perform a recently learnt task improves after six to eight hours' sleep. Without sleep, and without dreaming, you don't retain what you've learnt.

Improves your mood

Increased REM sleep also improves your mood. During sleep the brain makes serotonin. Both alcohol and many antidepressants suppress REM sleep. That's probably why you wake up grumpy if you go to sleep under the influence of alcohol. So, before you reach for the antidepressants, make sure you are getting enough sleep.

Regenerates and rejuvenates your body

Within half an hour of falling asleep, your body literally begins to rejuvenate itself. All through the night, and especially during deep sleep and REM phases, the brain produces higher levels of human growth hormone. This hormone helps with the repair and replacement of both tissue and bone. During the daytime, growth hormone levels are lower. When you're stressed, the subsequently high levels of the stress hormone cortisol further suppress growth hormone, diverting energy away from repair into coping with the energy demands of a stressful situation.

Normally when you are asleep, the levels of the stress hormone cortisol are low. But at times of chronic stress, cortisol levels may not drop sufficiently while you sleep. This further suppresses tissue repair, effectively speeding up the ageing process. This means that it's best to go to sleep unstressed. So horror movies last thing at night, or the late-night news, are bad news. Instead, do something relaxing and pleasant before going to sleep.

You live longer

The effects of sleep are far-reaching on your health. Both too little and too much are associated with an earlier death. Statistically, the amount of sleep that correlates with the longest lifespan is between five and nine hours a night. Particularly as we age, there is a higher correlation between few (less than five) and long (more than nine) hours of sleep and increased mortality. Seven hours' sleep is linked to the lowest death rate.[20] Just as important is the quality of sleep – many people, as they age, have more fragmented and light sleep and don't get enough time in slow wave or REM sleep.

How Much do You Need?

Before the invention of the electric light bulb, most people slept an average of 10 hours a night, especially in winter. By the 1960s, the average had dropped to eight hours. By 2000 the average was seven hours or less and now it continues to fall. More than one in three people get six hours or less. You need at least seven, and ideally eight, hours of good-quality, uninterrupted sleep to be healthy and happy.

How to Get a Good Night's Sleep

There are many factors that can disturb your sleep – noise, light and stimulants such as caffeine, to name only a few. Caffeine should be avoided for six hours before you sleep, as it lowers melatonin, which is the neurotransmitter that makes you sleepy in the evening. So, set yourself up for a good night's sleep. The more you balance your blood sugar level and deal with stress, the better you'll sleep.

If you don't sleep well, check your magnesium level. This relaxing mineral is in seeds, fruit and vegetables, especially dark green vegetables. Also try supplementing 300mg in the evening. If you need a little help getting to sleep try the herb kava (120mg of kavalactones) or the amino acid 5-HTP (100mg). Valerian is good too.

22

Sugar – Cut It Out

EATING SUGAR IS LIKE putting rocket fuel in a Mini – there's a quick burst of energy followed by a rapid burn-out. This is because the more sugar and refined carbohydrates you eat the more you become unable to maintain an even blood sugar level. The first symptoms of blood sugar problems include fatigue, irritability, poor concentration, forgetfulness, excessive thirst and low moods. One of the world's experts on blood sugar problems, Professor Gerald Reaven from Stanford University in California, estimates that one in four people show the early signs of losing blood sugar control. It's not a pretty picture.

Why It's Bad

- Sugar uses up your body's stores of vitamins and minerals and provides next to none. Every teaspoon of sugar uses up B vitamins, for example, which therefore makes you more deficient. B vitamins are vital for maximising your energy, both physically and mentally. About 98 per cent of the chromium present in sugar cane is lost in turning it into sugar. This mineral is vital for keeping your blood sugar level stable.

- Sugar makes you stupid. Researchers at the Massachusetts Institute of Technology found that the higher the intake of refined carbohydrates – such as sugar, commercial cereals, white bread and sweets – the lower the IQ. In fact, the difference between the high sugar consumers and the low sugar consumers was a staggering 25 points![21]

- Sugar makes you fat. This is because the more frequently your blood sugar is raised, the more insulin you produce. The more insulin you produce, the more sugar you dump as

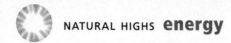

fat. Sugar can not only lead to weight gain and obesity, but also to water retention. If your body is too full of sugar, you'll retain excess fluid too, as every molecule of sugar will hold water.

- Eating too much sugar and refined carbohydrates not only zaps your energy; it also has many harmful effects on your health. Glucose is highly toxic. That's why the body tries to get it out of the blood as quickly as possible. Too much glucose damages the arteries, kidneys, eyes, brain and nerves, which is what often happens in people with diabetes. A high-sugar diet inflames the brain[22] and increases your risk of Alzheimer's later in life.

- Sugar can also upset your mood. Anyone who suffers from depression, PMS, hyperactivity, irritability, mood swings or angry outbursts should examine whether they are having a problem controlling their blood sugar.

- Sugar is best avoided completely. The trouble is, it's addictive. If you've become reliant on a daily intake of sugar or sweet foods, and if the thought of stopping them overnight makes you shudder, you may well want to take a look at the possibility of some level of an addiction.

You know you're a sugar addict if you lie about how much sweet food you have eaten; or keep a supply of sweet food close to hand; or hide it from others – and get upset if someone eats your supply; or go out of your way to get something sweet; or swoon at the dessert menu and always take a mint on the way out; or turn to sweets or chocolate whenever you're upset; or build sugary 'treats' into your day.

What's the Alternative?

The worst kinds of sugar are glucose, sucrose and dextrose. However, the sugar in honey and maple syrup isn't much different. These are all 'fast-releasing' sugars, which supply a quick burst of energy and a rapid burn-out. The sugar in most fruit is called fructose. This is 'slow-releasing' and therefore gives you more sustained energy, with less chance of throwing your blood sugar

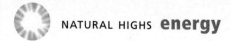

out of balance. What's more, fresh fruit contains many of the vitamins and minerals the body needs to turn glucose into energy.

So the alternative to sugar is fresh fruit. Some are better than others. Apples, pears and berries keep your blood sugar level most even because they are highest in fructose. Bananas, dates and raisins are higher in glucose-like sugars and are therefore best kept to a minimum. Having said that, if the choice is a Mars Bar or a banana, choose the banana. Eat fruit as snacks and sweeten your morning cereal or dinner-time dessert with fresh fruit.

How to Quit

Since sugar and the taste for sweet foods are addictive, it's best to wean yourself off them gradually. Cut those two spoonfuls of sugar in your tea to one for a week, then half a teaspoon for a week, then none. Whenever you crave something sweet, have a piece of fruit. It takes about a month to get used to having a no-sugar diet.

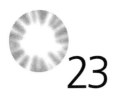

23

T'ai Chi

TAKE A STROLL through any city park in China and you are likely to see dozens of people calmly absorbed in a slow, graceful form of exercise. Millions of Chinese – from business executives to grandmothers – practise t'ai chi every day to maintain health and enhance energy levels. Now it's becoming increasingly popular in the West, especially for relieving stress.

What It Is

T'ai chi is a gentle form of exercise that helps you cultivate your chi or vital life force to become more energised. It involves performing a series of turning and stretching movements together with deep controlled breathing, which together refresh and stimulate your body without tiring you.

Although many practise it for its health benefits, t'ai chi is actually a martial art. But because of its meditative qualities, it's also called Chinese yoga. And like yoga, there are many schools of t'ai chi – Chen, Wu, Taoist and Sun are some of the most common – but the most popular in the West is Yang.

Each style has its unique features, but all teach a series of movements starting from an upright position that connect into a harmonised sequence called 'the form'. Every movement flows into the next and requires you to relax rather than tense differ- ent muscle groups, a process that opens up your joints to increase energy flow and circulation. As you progress, you can add more movements to create a longer form, but most routines last around 7 to 10 minutes.

Breathing is an essential part of t'ai chi. Learning to control your breath is what helps relax and energise you. When you can do this, you can then start to feel your *chi* flow into your hands and throughout your body.

Why It's Good

Regular practice increases physical stamina and flexibility and helps bring a sense of inner calm, as well as improving health and vitality. Advocates claim that it's an effective therapy for a wide range of medical conditions, including poor circulation, high blood pressure, arthritis, back pain, breathing difficulties and digestive and nervous disorders. In China, doctors even prescribe it as a form of treatment.

You don't have to be particularly fit or flexible to learn t'ai chi. Anyone of any age can do it, and the degree of exertion can be easily adjusted to suit each individual. Ageing doesn't decrease ability either – someone of 70 can be just as accomplished or even better than a 25-year-old.

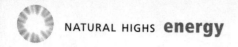

How to Learn It

Although there are videos you can buy, the most effective way is to attend a class where you can follow an instructor. They can help you perfect the movements that make up the form. Your posture and breathing during each movement needs to be as exact as possible to get the most benefit.

Once you know the physical moves and you don't have to think about where you are going to put your foot or arm next, it becomes second nature and you can concentrate on relaxing. Using the breathing, you can then start to focus on your chi or life force to become more energised.

You don't need any special equipment to do t'ai chi – just a smooth floor space, comfortable clothing and shoes that provide good support and balance. Once you've learnt the basics, you can practise the movements and breathing at home in addition to, or instead of, attending a weekly class.

For information on how to find a class, see Resources on page 147.

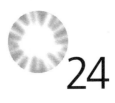

24

Think Positive!

SOME PEOPLE ALWAYS notice what's wrong, and complain about it. Others notice what's right and do something about what isn't. As the famous Serenity Prayer reads: 'Give me the strength to change the things I can, the patience to accept that which I cannot change, and the wisdom to know the difference.'

Thinking positively is a habit, and a good one to develop. It keeps you energised and motivated. Here's how.

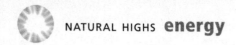

Create your own reality

Give yourself permission to dream, then make your dreams come true. Visualise what you want to happen, when you are in a deep state of relaxation or meditation, perhaps before you go to sleep or when you wake up. People who make things happen have dreams, share their dreams and take the steps necessary for the dreams to come true. Ask yourself: 'What do I need to do for this dream to come true?' Then do it.

Focus on what you can do – and do it

In any situation, ask yourself what contribution you can make – and make it. Notice what works and, where other people are concerned, acknowledge them for that, and do something about the stuff that doesn't, rather than just complaining about it. George Bernard Shaw once said, 'Everyone complains about the weather but nobody does anything about it.'

Ask what you can give, not what you can get

In any situation focus on what you can offer, perhaps at work or in a relationship. It is a universal law that the more you give the more you receive. Don't give expecting to receive. You'll always be disappointed. One of our favourite sayings is, 'No good deed goes unpunished.' It helps you to stay focused on unconditional giving.

Give yourself fully to whatever you are doing

There's no point in doing something in a half-hearted way. It just isn't as much fun. If you commit to something, commit to it 100 per cent. If you commit to a relationship 70 per cent, and your partner does the same, 70 per cent of 70 per cent is 49 per cent. That's a failure.

'Never' or 'always' means a negative pattern

When you find yourself saying to someone, 'You never . . .' or 'You always . . .', you can bet that the person's behaviour is touching something unresolved in your past. It could involve a parent who used to say to you, 'You never . . .' or 'You always . . .' When you find yourself reacting strongly and almost automatically to someone's behaviour in this way, take some time to reflect on any similar patterns in your own past history.

Count your blessings

Literally do it. When you find yourself thinking that nothing is working right in your life, stop and count all your blessings. Notice everything you have, everything you've learnt, all your blessings. Be grateful for what you have and change what you haven't. As one meditation master, Swami Muktananda, said, 'The world is as you see it. Change the prescription of your glasses.'

If you've got something to do, do it

Start your day by doing something big. Getting a 'result' early in the day keeps you positive. There's a rhyme that goes, 'Procrastination, she said, was the source of all my sorrow. I don't know what that word means. I'll look it up tomorrow.'

Make a mistake, and learn from it, every day

We learn by making mistakes. Instead of giving yourself a hard time every time you make a mistake, acknowledge that you learn by making mistakes. Ask yourself how you could have done that better, and do it better next time. The past is history.

Say how you feel and move on

It is natural to sometimes be sad, angry or fearful. Don't deny your feelings. If someone asks how you are, don't just say, 'I'm fine.' Tell them how you *really* feel. This will help you to have some perspective on your feelings, which inevitably change, rather than being all caught up in them. When you allow yourself to feel, and express your feelings, you may be surprised by what you feel. Behind sadness is often anger. As one person once said, 'Depression is anger without enthusiasm.' If you hang on to negative feelings, they stay with you forever. If you don't deny them, they inevitably wither up and blow away. This is easier said than done, and may mean forgiving someone for something they did to you. The question you have to ask yourself is, 'Do you want to be right, or do you want to be happy?' Suppressed feelings deplete both your happiness and your energy.

25

Yoga – Enlighten Your Body

IF YOU OFTEN find yourself feeling not just tired, but dispirited and somehow disconnected from life and those around you, let yoga transform you. A good yoga class is uplifting, exhilarating and rejuvenating. Whether you're practising yoga more for body than soul, or vice-versa, you can guarantee that every time you do yoga, you'll be regenerating the whole you: mind, body and spirit.

Yet in the West, many of us still tend to regard yoga purely as a form of physical exercise. In fact, yoga is the ancient Indian science and practice of obtaining freedom and liberation. The physical exercises of hatha yoga are only one branch of this science, in which breath, movement and posture are harmonised to remove physical and emotional blocks and tension and re-energise the body.

Why It's Good

Hatha yoga tones the muscles, improves flexibility and gets your body fighting fit. As pure exercise, it's a natural high in itself, improving your circulation and oxygenating the blood, making you feel energised and more 'alive'. It also stimulates the release of endorphins, boosting your mood and bringing a feeling of euphoria. But yoga brings you benefits that reach far beyond those you would get from an aerobic class or a jog around the park. Research shows that yoga has positive effects on pulse, blood pressure, and mental and physical performance beyond those expected from physical exercise alone.

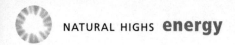

A stress-buster and natural high

As I've mentioned, the body accumulates blockages in the form of tension. These blockages prevent vital energy – known in India as *prana* – from restoring your vitality. As we accumulate stresses throughout the day, these get stored away as anxiety in our minds and as tension in our bodies. The more anxious and tense we feel, the less energised we become. Regular yoga practice releases any stored-up tension and keeps your body relaxed and your mind calm.

More energy, more relaxation

Yoga engages the body, the breath and the mind, uniting all three to bring you to a natural and blissful state of equilibrium. In fact, the word yoga comes from the Sanskrit word for 'union'. Often described as 'meditation in action', yoga brings you clarity of mind, relaxation and increased energy and alertness.

It's amazingly versatile

The beauty of yoga is that anyone can do it. Whether you're an Olympic athlete or an expectant mother, you can tailor your yoga practice to suit your fitness level and lifestyle. Yoga can also be used to relieve pain and help in the treatment of specific injuries. If you have a specific ailment or injury, ask a qualified yoga teacher to advise you on a remedial programme.

Finding the Right Kind

There are several different schools of hatha yoga that you can choose from. Iyengar yoga is a precise, slow form that focuses on posture to help realign the body so the vital energy can flow properly. Astanga yoga is more athletic and physically demanding. Both forms will leave you feeling more relaxed and energised, but some people naturally prefer Astanga yoga, while others respond best to Iyengar. Try them both and see what suits you.

Although you can buy books or videos on yoga, by far the best and safest way to learn is to find a class near you (see

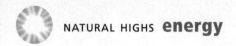

below for how to obtain a list of schools). Once you've learnt the postures, you can practice yoga at home, perhaps accompanied by some relaxing or energising music.

Any Precautions?

Even though yoga is relatively low-impact and safe, physical injury is still possible if undertaken without proper instruction. Be sure to seek the advice of a fully qualified yoga teacher before beginning your yoga practice. Also, let them know of any specific injury or illness you may have.

Where to Find It

See Resources on page 147 for information on finding a teacher or class in your area.

144

Notes

1 J. B. Deijin et al., 'Tyrosine improves cognitive performance and reduces blood pressure in cadets', *Brain Research Bulletin*, Vol. 48(2) (1999), pp. 203–9.

2 D. Benton and G. Roberts, 'Effect of vitamin and mineral supplementation on intelligence of school children', *The Lancet*, Vol.1(8578) (1988), pp. 140–3.

3 N. J. Richardson, P. J. Rogers et al., 'Mood and performance effects of caffeine in relation to acute and chronic caffeine deprivation', *Pharmacology Biochemistry and Behavior*, Vol. 52(2), (1995), pp. 313–20.

4 K. Gilliland and D. Andress, 'Ad lib caffeine consumption, symptoms of caffeinism, and academic performance', *American Journal of Psychiatry*, Vol. 138(4) (1981), pp. 512–4.

5 A. E. Hunt et al., 'Effect of chromium supplementation on hair chromium concentration and diabetic status', *Nutr Res*, Vol. 5 (1985), pp. 131–40.

6 R. A. Anderson et al., 'Chromium supplementation of humans with hypoglycaemia', *Fed Proc*, Vol. 43 (1984), p. 471.

7 G. Evans, 'The effect of chromium picolinate on insulin controlled parameters in humans', *Int J Biosocial and Med Research*, Vol. 1(2) (1989), pp. 163–80.

8 S. Davies et al., 'Age-related decreases in chromium levels in 51,665 hair, sweat and serum samples from 40,872 patients – implications for the prevention of cardiovascular disease and type II diabetes mellitus', *Metabolism*, Vol. 46(5) (1997), pp. 1–4.

9 D. Lobstein et al., 'Beta-endorphin and components of emotionality discriminate between physically active and sedentary men', *Biol Psychiatry*, Vol. 26(1) (May 1989), pp. 3–14.

10 W. McArdle, (chapter in) *Medical Aspects of Clinical Nutrition*, Keats Publishing (1983).

11 D. Broughton et al., 'Deterioration of glucose tolerance with age: the role of insulin resistance', *Age and Ageing*, Vol. 20 (1991), pp. 221–5.

12 C. Hollenbeck et al., 'Effect of habitual exercise on regulation of insulin stimulated glucose disposal in older males', *J Am Geriatr Soc*, Vol. 33 (1986), pp. 273–7.

13 Farnsworth et al., 'Siberian ginseng: current status as an adaptogen', in H. Wagner et al. (eds.), *Economic and Medicinal Plant Research 1*, Academic Press (1985), pp.156–215.

14 E. Ploss, 'Panax ginseng', *Kooperation Phytopharmaka* (1988); and U. Sonnenborn and Y. Proppert 'Panax ginseng', *Z. Phytoptherapie*, Vol. 11 (1990), pp. 35–49. Both papers are quoted in V. Schultz et al., *Rational Phytotherapy*, Springer (1998).

15 D. Rosen, *Green Tea: Good Health in Your Cup*, Souvenir Press (1998).

16 M. A. MacKenzie et al., 'The influence of glycyrrhetinic acid on plasma cortisol and cortisone in healthy young volunteers', *J Clin Endocrinol Metab*, Vol. 70(6) (1990), pp. 1637–43.

17 C. Germano and Z. Ramazanov, *Arctic Root (Rhodiola rosea)*, Kensington Books (1999).

18 A. A. Spasov et al., 'A double-blind, placebo-controlled pilot study of the stimulating and adaptogenic effect of *Rhodiola rosea* SHR-5 extract on the fatigue of students caused by stress during an examination period with a repeated low-dose regimen', *Phytomedicine*, Vol. 7(2), (2000), pp. 85–9.

19 R. Stickgold et al., 'Sleep, learning, and dreams: off-line memory reprocessing', *Science*, Vol. 294(5544) (2001), pp. 1052–7.

20 D. L. Wingard et al., 'A multivariate analysis of health-related practices: a nine-year mortality follow-up of the Alameda County Study', *Am J Epidemiol*, Vol. 116(5) (1982), pp. 765–75.

21 A. G. Shauss, 'Nutrition and behavior', *Journal of Applied Nutrition*, Vol. 35(1) (1983), pp. 30–5; and proceedings of MIT conference on Research Strategies for Assessing the Behavioural Effects of Foods and Nutrients (1982).

22 F. G. Epstein, 'Mechanisms of disease', *N Eng J Med*, Vol. 334(6) (1996), pp. 374–81.

Resources

For further information about topics covered in *Natural Highs Energy*, see our book *Natural Highs*.

Chapter 10

UK: Training videos and further details are available from P/Cals UK, PO Box 388, Wembley HA9 9GP. Or you can call 020 8728 0211, fax 020 8930 7311 or email info@pcals-uk.com.

Overseas readers: Overseas readers can order training videos and ask for further information through P/Cals UK, address as above or found on the web at www.pcals.com. You can find details of teachers in your local area by contacting the Arica Institute, PO Box 645, Kent, CT 06757 USA, phone 1 860 927 1006 or email office@arica.org. The Institute holds the worldwide register of Psychocalisthenics teachers.

Chapter 16

UK: Two courses that have received good feedback are the one-day Learn to Meditate courses offered by Siddha Yoga, and courses at the London Buddhist Centre. Both groups have regional networks and can be contacted at: Siddha Yoga Meditation Centre, 32 Cubitt Street, London WC1X 0LR, or call 020 7278 0035. The London

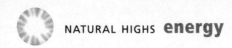

Buddhist Centre can be reached at 51 Roman Road, London E2 0HU, or call 020 8981 1225.

Australia: The Siddha Yoga Foundation Australia holds training courses throughout Australia in capital cities and regional centres. Their website is www.siddhayoga.org.au.

New Zealand: For Siddha Yoga centres in New Zealand visit www.siddhayoga.org. Also try www.nzhealth.net.nz/nzregister/ meditate.html or www.buddhanet.net/nzbudir2.htm for listings of meditation and Buddhist meditation centres and teachers through-out New Zealand.

Singapore: For Siddha Yoga centres in Singapore visit www.siddhayoga.org. Or, for Buddhist meditation, contact the Odiyana Buddhist Meditation Centre, Singapore: www.meditateinsingapore.org.

South Africa: For Siddha Yoga centres in South Africa visit www.siddhayoga.org. Buddhanet lists a variety of Buddhist medita-tion centres throughout South Africa: their website is www.buddhanet.net/africame/africadir.htm.

Chapter 18

For details of training or to arrange one-to-one or small group trainings, contact MetaFitness, Squire's Hill House, Tilford, Surrey GU10 2AD. You can call them on 01252 782661.

Self-tuition kits are available from P/CALS UK, PO Box 388, Wembley HA9 9GP, or call 020 8728 0211, fax 020 8930 7311 or email info@pcals-uk.com. Further information about Psychocalisthenics can be found on www.pcals.com.

Training courses are not available in Australia, New Zealand, Singapore or South Africa, but training videos and further information are available from www.pcals.com.

Chapter 24

UK: For more information or to find out about classes in your area, contact the T'ai Chi Union for Great Britain, 1 Littlemill Drive, Balmoral Gardens, Crookston, Glasgow G53 7GE, or call 0141 810 3482. The Taoist T'ai Chi Society of Great Britain also runs classes around the UK. Contact them at Bounstead Road, Blackheath, Colchester, Essex CO2 0DE, or call 01206 576167. If you're London-based, try the London School of T'ai Chi Chuan and Traditional Health Resources at PO Box 9836, London SE3 0ZG, or call 07626 914 540.

Overseas readers: You can find out about local classes by asking at local alternative health centres or health food shops. Also check in the telephone directory under sports clubs and associations, complementary therapies or martial arts.

Chapter 25

UK: The British Wheel of Yoga can put you in touch with a yoga school or teacher in your area (call 01529 303 233). So can the Iyengar Yoga Institute, Maida Vale, London W9 1NL. Call them on 020 7624 3080 or visit their website, iyi.org.uk.

Australia: The Siddha Yoga Foundation Australia teaches yoga throughout Australia in capital cities and regional centres. Their website is www.siddhayoga.org.au.

New Zealand: A list of registered yoga teachers and centres throughout New Zealand can be found at the New Zealand Register of Complementary Health Professionals: www.nzhealth.net. nz/nzregister/yoga_nz.html.

Singapore: Hatha Yoga is taught at the various Sports for Life Centres throughout Singapore. Email ssc_spa@ssc.gov.sg for more details.

South Africa: Find an Iyengar Yoga teacher at this website: www.bksiyengar.co.za/html/teacherslist.html.

Visit **www.naturallyhigh.co.uk**
for up-to-date information on:

- The latest natural highs products and suppliers
- The latest articles, research and information on legal, natural, mind-altering substances
- Your questions answered
- Natural highs seminars and workshops near you
- Natural highs books, CDs and other resources.

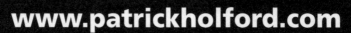